ENGAGING PHYSICIANS

A MANUAL TO PHYSICIAN PARTNERSHIP

"Dr. Beeson's new book couldn't have come at a better time. His step-by-step approach to achieving powerful collaboration with physicians is the perfect prescription for what is needed to deliver on the promise of clinically excellent and compassionate care. This new manual should be required reading for all healthcare executives and physician leaders who aspire to create a better future for their patients and themselves."

—David S. Fox, President, Advocate Good Samaritan Hospital

"Dr. Beeson skillfully and systematically lays out a road map for empowering physicians to lead the change in healthcare delivery. This proven methodology provides the structure and skills for physicians to hold each other accountable for providing excellent care. This book is a must-read for physician and healthcare organization leaders who wish to take charge in creating systems of safe, efficient, and effective care. The kind of care you want for yourself and your family."

—Ken Davis, MD, Chief Medical Officer,
San Antonio Methodist Healthcare System

"Engaging Physicians *fills the gap created by* Hardwiring Excellence *and* Practicing Excellence, *serving as a 'how-to' manual to guide practices in their efforts to build a culture of service excellence. Dr. Beeson, with his vast experience in medical system organizational change in his own Sharp Experience, as well as nationally through his coaching, lays out step-by-step the methods to inspire physician engagement. He also provides the tools organizations will need to train physicians to improve the quality and service of the healthcare they deliver to every patient, every time."*

—William Storo, MD, Pediatrician, Dartmouth Hitchcock, Concord, NH

ENGAGING PHYSICIANS

A MANUAL TO PHYSICIAN PARTNERSHIP

Stephen C. Beeson, MD

Published by:
Fire Starter Publishing
913 Gulf Breeze Parkway, Suite 6
Gulf Breeze, FL 32561
Phone: 850-934-1099
Fax: 850-934-1384
www.firestarterpublishing.com

ISBN: 978-0-9840794-0-7

Library of Congress Control Number: 2009929133

Printed in the United States of America

Table of Contents

Foreword

Here are some of the most frequently asked questions and statements I have received from healthcare leaders:

- "How do we engage the medical staff?"
- "Are the physicians going to do this?"
- "What about the doctors? You know their behavioral issues."
- "Our biggest challenge is the physicians. They are not loyal to the organization. They keep moving profitable services to their offices."

Here are the most often asked questions and statements I hear from physicians:

- "You would think they would ask us what we think."
- "How can they do this when they can't even get the nurses to have the charts when they call me?"
- "Why don't they hold people accountable?"
- "How come no one says anything to me when things are going well? The only time I hear from administration is when there is a problem or they want something."
- "Why do they keep wasting money on consultants and programs? I can tell them what they need to do."
- "The only ones who get treated well around here are the surgeons because they bring in the money."
- "They favor the docs they employ versus us, the independent physicians."

- "Wish they would ask *me* sometime. I have given hours of free time to the hospital with little thanks for it."

I see organizations where there is excellent collaboration between the organization and the medical staff. I also see the consequences when good alignment is not present. When physician partnership is in place, patient care is better, staff enjoys work more, and the physicians find a much more effective and efficient place to take care of patients, conduct research, or provide their diagnostic skills. When this happens administration enjoys their work more, the organization performs well, and the quality of life in the entire system improves.

The question is *How do leaders build a collaborative, cooperative relationship with physicians that earns physician loyalty and engages physicians to work toward a shared agenda?*

Dr. Beeson has followed up his best-selling first book, *Practicing Excellence*, geared for practicing physicians in office settings, with his newest book, *Engaging Physicians: A Manual to Physician Partnership*. This book will answer the challenging and repetitive questions leaders have about "getting physicians on board" and build the structure to align physicians in a mutually beneficial partnership. Written by a physician, the book is loaded with treatment plans and prescriptions on how to best gain collaboration for excellent care.

In the last four years, Dr. Beeson has had the opportunity to facilitate Studer Group sessions for healthcare leaders, present and teach in organizations, and harvest best practices throughout the country. He also interacts often with Studer Group coaches in their work. This work, combined with his work and leadership role in his medical group, has given him the unique experience of seeing life on both sides of the fence.

His book *Engaging Physicians: A Manual to Physician Partnership* shows how to take the fence down and keep it down. Today's healthcare environment is tough, and organizations that execute in quality, safety, and service will win. Most organizations do not have the time or resources to waste that comes from physicians and administrators moving in different directions and pursuing different goals. Dr. Beeson has become a specialist in helping leaders work with physicians in a genuine spirit of "win/win," where physicians, the organization, and patients all benefit.

I met Dr. Beeson through our work with his organization. In our early work with the system, our work was moving too fast for some and way too slow for physicians. Lesson one: Physicians' and non-physicians' sense of time are vastly different. What is quick to a non-physician can appear slow to a physician.

One day I received a call that Sharp Rees-Stealy Medical Group had appointed a physician to lead the work to hardwire excellence and would be attending the Taking You and Your Organization to the Next Level training session. Dr. Beeson's attendance helped impact his own practice with the Sharp Rees-Stealy Medical Group, where patient satisfaction increased from the 13th to the 89th percentile during the time of his appointment.

With the success of his work, organizations requested to learn more. To that end, Studer Group created a Physician Institute for physicians. Dr. Beeson is one of our lead facilitators. He also wrote *Practicing Excellence*, which has sold over 50,000 copies to-date, to help physicians provide better care to patients. He speaks across the country to some of the best healthcare systems in the country on physician engagement and physician performance improvement.

With this book, Dr. Beeson reaches out again to make healthcare better. Dr. Beeson could easily present on his work and do very well financially. But he chooses to limit these for now to stay close to his two loves: his family and his patients. After these two loves, he makes time for a third one: the desire to make the quality of life better for physicians, staff, patients, and their families.

Quint Studer

This book is dedicated to my wife, Deanna, and kids, Sydney and Nicholas, who made sacrifices and patiently supported me while I wrote this manuscript.

I also dedicate this book to physicians across the nation as they rediscover the greatness of our profession and rekindle the fire of making a difference in the lives of patients.

Introduction

Sometimes we end up in places we didn't plan to go. That certainly has been the case for me. I am a practicing family medicine physician with the Sharp Rees-Stealy Medical Group in San Diego, California, where I have maintained an active clinical practice for the last 15 years. I am married to my beautiful wife, Deanna, and am the father of two amazing kids, Sydney and Nicholas, who are 12 and 10 at the time of this writing. Practicing medicine and raising a family were the parts of my life that I had planned.

The part of my life that I didn't plan began in 2002. Sharp HealthCare, made up of four hospitals and three medical groups, including Sharp Rees-Stealy, launched a systemwide effort to transform the healthcare experience for employees, physicians, and patients. We called our effort "The Sharp Experience."

Prior to this new organizational commitment, we had considered ourselves the leader in our competitive marketplace, and certainly a very good integrated system by most standards. In an effort to get a more precise "state of the system," Sharp HealthCare leadership wanted to dig deeper to find out how things were going at the front line. Focus groups were conducted involving staff, physicians, and patients to find out how we rated as a place for employees to work, physicians to practice medicine, and patients to receive care. Though the results were "okay," we were clearly not as good as we thought we were. Something different needed to be done, and the search for a change strategy began.

In 2000, after an intensive cross-country search and significant due diligence, Sharp HealthCare partnered with Studer Group, a healthcare outcomes firm with a proven record of transformational results. The goal of the partnership was to execute a cultural shift and take Sharp HealthCare to the next level.

Goals were established, leadership was developed, staff was trained, strategies were formulated, and action plans were initiated. Despite vigorous initial efforts, the deeply seeded culture of "we are pretty good" was more challenging to shift. Our burning platform for change was lukewarm, at best. Being "pretty good" was never the ambition of Sharp HealthCare or any members of our leadership team. The first year of the Sharp Experience yielded minimal improvement and was certainly not the "transformation" that was the intention of our new organizational commitment.

One year after the launch of the Sharp Experience, with little change in our performance measures, an annual employee opinion survey was conducted to take the pulse of the workforce. The result of the survey provided us a diagnostic glimpse into our struggles. The leading dissatisfier for our employees was not pay, work conditions, benefits, or complaints about "administration." The most important and lowest performing issue for our employees was the conduct and behavior of our physicians. Our front line employees were frustrated with physicians not doing what the rest of the staff was trained and required to do. They asked, "If the Sharp Experience is so important, and we are held to such high standards, why aren't the physicians doing it?" Physicians were not included in the launch of the Sharp Experience because the leadership team wanted to get our "house in order" prior to getting physicians involved. We began to realize we had made a strategic error.

We significantly underestimated the impact of the "non-engaged," uninvolved physician. We coached and trained staff members who would spend much of their day interacting with physicians who had little working knowledge, awareness, or support of the "mission" of the system. Our staff saw physicians as the leaders of the clinical care team, and they would do as they saw their leaders do. We trained our staff in a new commitment to service excellence, while our physicians continued in the old way of doing things. The impact and sustainability of service training efforts were lost as our staff gravitated to the conduct of physicians. Physicians became unknowing obstructionists to system change based on a failure to access their partnership, support, and leadership.

The awareness of physicians' influence on our staff was one thing. Doing something about it was something else, entirely. For the Sharp Experience to work, our leadership team realized that physician alignment, engagement, and participation had to happen. We needed a strategy to reach our physicians to make them part of the collective effort. Our team was also keenly aware that administrators standing in front of physicians and asking them to "get on the bus" was not going to work. The message of the Sharp Experience needed to come from a physician as a colleague-to-colleague gesture. It was becoming clear that a new physician position was in evolution. That is when the unplanned part of my life began.

In 2002, I was appointed by our board of directors to be the physician champion for the Sharp Experience. My directives were to bring the Sharp Experience to physicians, and to clarify and train the physician role in a systemwide effort. Our goals were to create physician involvement and support for the Sharp Experience and to improve physician performance in quality and service. I was tasked with the daunting challenge of creating physician behavior change and generating physician loyalty to a broad, grassroots change strategy.

After a slow and difficult beginning, the Sharp Experience journey was beginning to work. We coached, trained, measured, benchmarked, and partnered with physicians to achieve our goals. Results in patient satisfaction and quality began to materialize as physicians and staff worked together to improve patient care. Patients were noticing, and a sense of pride and accomplishment began to spread throughout the organization. The Sharp Experience was transforming who we were, and began to unify our workforce to achieve something extraordinary. The Sharp Experience became our identity, our signature, and what we became known for in the community.

In 2007, we gained national recognition by winning the Malcolm Baldrige Quality Award. Two of the Sharp Hospitals, including our main Memorial Campus, and the Cabrillo Nursing Facility received Magnet designation by the American Nursing Credentialing Center for excellence in nursing practice and patient care. In the same year, the Sharp Rees-Stealy Medical Group was an honoree recipient of the prestigious American Medical Group Association Acclaim Award. In 2008, Sharp Rees-Stealy was ranked the number one group in the state of California in clinical quality and the patient experience for the third consecutive year, a ranking compiled by health plans rating over 200 systems.

I had the opportunity to meet with healthcare leaders who were embarking on similar journeys and were challenged by the prospect of getting physicians engaged. I heard the same questions, frustrations, obstacles, and concerns from clinic, hospital, and emergency room leaders from across the country. Leaders realized that physician participation was a key to effective change, but solid guidance on this front was sparse. I wanted to help. I wanted to be a part of making healthcare better and to help foster system and physician partnerships so patients would benefit.

In 2005, I was invited to serve as a medical director for Studer Group. I received requests from systems across the country to coach and train physicians to improve clinical and service performance. Though physician morale has been under assault on a national scale, I found hope, optimism, and aspiration from physicians everywhere I went. Physicians wanted to be better, and were willing to lead the way. It was an intense and promising time, and I began to compile the strategies that were working to improve physician performance.

In 2006, I wrote *Practicing Excellence: A Physician's Manual to Exceptional Health Care.* My purpose was to provide physicians guidance to improve the care provided to patients and the work environment they created for themselves and their staff. *Practicing Excellence* was written to help physicians be professionally successful by providing training and skills that every physician needs but very few receive.

Though *Practicing Excellence* was written to improve physician performance, it left many questions unanswered and challenges unaddressed. As I spoke with healthcare leaders, I heard consistent and recurrent challenges. How do we get physicians involved? How do we restore physician loyalty to our hospital? How do we get physicians to care about what we are doing? How do we appoint a physician champion? What does a physician champion do? How do we improve patient satisfaction with our affiliated medical staff? What do we do when physicians vocally protest change efforts? How do we create strategies where physicians and hospitals work hard to achieve goals together? These recurrent leader challenges were the inspiration for this book.

Engaging Physicians: A Manual to Physician Partnership will take leaders on a stepwise, staged journey to engage physicians in a systemwide effort and align physician behavior to achieve worthy, evidence-based organizational goals. *Engaging Physicians* begins with Stage 1, "Create and Communicate Organizational Vision and Goals." This stage takes leaders through the creation of a compelling organizational vision that is boldly projected throughout the organization. Clarity of direction and communication of vision are requirements for enrolling physicians in a unified, shared agenda. Workforce unity will determine the success of change efforts.

Stage 2, "Leadership Development and Accountability for Performance," is a guide to assembling a high-performance leadership structure, built to achieve outcomes based on a proven "evidence-based leadership" model. Effective leaders who do as they say and execute outcomes earn the respect and loyalty of physicians. A high-performing leadership team with a track record of performance builds credibility, a prerequisite to physician engagement.

Stage 3, "Establishing Physician Confidence and Trust," is a specific guide to creating the facility of choice for physicians. By delivering a best-in-class physician experience, physician receptiveness and willingness to participate in the shared agenda are created.

Stage 4, "Building Physician Leadership," progresses to developing an effective and aligned physician leadership structure including the traditional structural leadership team, as well as the role of physician champions.

Stage 5, "Training Physicians," is about investing in the medical staff using a proven physician training model. An organization that helps and supports physicians through evidence-based training is a powerful alignment strategy by clarifying physicians' roles in the organizational effort and providing worthy guidance to make them more successful.

Stage 6, "Physician Measurement and Balanced Scorecards," instructs leaders on performance feedback and data reporting to drive and improve outcomes delivered by physicians. If properly applied, performance feedback can be one of the most effective physician improvement and behavioral change strategies.

Stage 7, "Implementing Physician Behavioral Standards," is about the creation, implementation and communication of behavioral standards currently required by the Joint Commissions.

Stage 8, "Managing the Disruptive Physician," provides specific leader guidance on managing violations of a code of conduct, historically one of the most dreaded and poorly performed leadership activities.

Stage 9, "Recognizing Physicians," provides simple tactics to recognize physicians. Physician recognition remains one of the most important drivers of physician satisfaction and is a high-yield activity for building physician relationships with the organization and its leadership team.

Engaging Physicians: A Manual to Physician Partnership is a distilled method of changing physician behavior and creating willingness, and even enthusiasm, to participate in system-based care. The independent, isolated physician's renting of a hospital room to care for patients was done yesterday. Today and tomorrow are about physician partnership, collaboration, and leadership to deliver evidence-based medicine, superior outcomes, and exceptional service where nurses, physicians, and administration work together to achieve shared goals.

The process of engaging physicians is among the most important strategies to transform healthcare performance. Physicians will make or break the culture, performance, and reputation of the institution and can accelerate or unravel quality, safety, and service efforts. Physician participation in a system effort is based upon factors and conditions that many healthcare leaders fail to realize, and these well-intentioned leaders can wonder in utter frustration why physicians do the things they do.

Physicians are selective and deliberate in engaging in an organizational change strategy. In the end, physicians will do for the organization what the organization has done for them. Physicians will partner with administration when trust and confidence in the leadership team are built, clinical efficiency is demonstrated, and physicians have meaningful input on organizational efforts. When physician alliance is created, physicians will be an organization's greatest champions, will expect more of themselves, will recruit their colleagues, will appoint physicians who align with the mission, and will leverage their influence to change culture. The highest performing healthcare systems in the country are led by engaged, aligned physicians who work passionately and collaboratively to implement superior, evidence-based care and extraordinary service as a unified commitment.

Physicians and health system leaders want the same things. We depend on each other to achieve our mission to improve care for our patients and improve the work experience for our staff and ourselves. Let's go on this journey to get this done.

STAGE 1:

CREATE AND COMMUNICATE ORGANIZATIONAL VISION AND GOALS

"Good leaders create a vision, articulate the vision, passionately own the vision, and relentlessly drive it to completion."

— Jack Welch

THE VISION

The crafting of an organizational vision is commonplace. The mere presence of a vision created in a strategy session and framed on a wall is not what differentiates one healthcare system from another. The measure of an organizational vision is never the content of its words, but its influence on those tasked to carry it out.

When I initially meet with physicians for health systems, I will ask them to articulate the vision of the organization. I ask physicians, "What is the organization trying to become?" It is alarmingly common to have physicians stare blankly back, with little awareness as to what they are trying to do. How can members of the team execute a strategy if they haven't been given the playbook? How can leadership lead physicians if the destination is not laser sharp, thoroughly communicated, agreed upon, and understood by everyone? How can the foundation to organizational change be passed over so commonly and so flagrantly?

Getting physicians on board *must* begin with clear and deliberate communication of the vision of the organization. Leaders must effectively and boldly project a credible, articulate destination that is better than current operations. Leader communication with physicians is not about a voice of authority mandating change, but rather a persuasive and compelling case that a different way of providing care will be better. A new organizational vision and case for change must be bound by logic and overwhelming evidence to generate physician support and minimize protest. Great leaders go beyond a simple strategic argument for organizational transformation. Great leaders know it will take more than persuasion to fully enroll physicians in visionary change. Great leaders create a shared vision that connects to the hopes, dreams, and aspirations of physicians and the entire healthcare workforce to make a difference, save lives, and be a part of something extraordinary.

Several years ago, I had a chance to meet David Barbe, M.D., president of St. John's Regional Division in Missouri. St. John's is an integrated healthcare system that consistently ranks as one of the highest performing systems in the country in patient satisfaction, with clear support, partnership, and engagement of their physicians. I asked Dr. Barbe how they became so successful. He told me that before St. John's initiated any change efforts, the leadership team invited physician stakeholders to sit at the table. Leaders clearly articulated a compelling case for the future and shared a vision for what they thought the organization could become. They asked for physician input and shared open dialogue to build consensus on St. John's direction, vision, and goals. They created physician buy-in "up-front" and repeated their transformational change strategy over and over, so all members of the medical staff and the entire healthcare system understood future plans. The leadership team worked diligently to secure consensus and awareness before implementing any of their strategic plans. They created a buzz about the upcoming leader commitments and the bright future awaiting St. John's.

The benefit and leverage of the vision for St. John's were less about its content than about how it was communicated. Physicians' awareness, understanding, and early involvement facilitated the system's change efforts. In fact, the same St. John's strategy, without proactive communication of vision and goals, may have provoked an entirely different physician response. When physicians are unaware, uninvolved, and kept in the dark, leaders should not be surprised to see indifference or rejection to an otherwise sound strategy.

I coached Dartmouth-Hitchcock Medical Center in New Hampshire in 2008. At the launch of their system's efforts, they shut down clinic operations for a half-day so that each of their physicians could attend a half-day training session. Dr. Cherie Holmes, an orthopedic surgeon and the Dartmouth medical director, spoke to the entire medical staff to convey the depth of the system's commitment and vision as to what Dartmouth could become. She communicated strategies and tactics to achieve system goals. Physicians left knowing exactly where the organization was going, how it intended to get there, and what role *they* played in a systemwide commitment to be the best. When physicians heard the vision, strategy, and goals from leaders they trusted and respected, the foundation for engagement and partnership was laid.

In 2007, Sharp HealthCare won the Malcolm Baldrige Award for organizational performance. It is the highest organizational honor in any industry and we were overwhelmed with pride that the hard work to change service, quality, and culture was paying off. I had a chance to be interviewed by Baldrige examiners. They listened intently as our leaders reviewed how we created and executed our vision. While they realized the leader level of our organization had a thorough grasp of the strategies and goals of Sharp HealthCare, what they most wanted to know was how the vision of the Sharp Experience had impacted our front line staff and practicing physicians. The beacon and guiding light of our organization was to become the best place for patients to receive care, the best place for physicians to practice medicine, and the best place for employees to work. The Baldrige evaluation of Sharp HealthCare was whether our mission was *embraced* by hourly employees, employed physicians, and the affiliated medical staff.

What good is a vision if it has little impact on those who are tasked to execute it? Does a vision even exist if it does not guide the daily actions of each member of the team? The Baldrige examiners assessed the credibility of our organizational strategy by the reach of our vision. The diffusion and projection of an organizational vision are a measure of leadership and remain as important as the vision itself.

Guidelines to Creating an Effective Organizational Vision:

1. **Invite and include physician leadership, practicing physicians, and staff to participate in creation of the organizational vision.** Input to change efforts in systems paves the way for receptiveness to change. When physicians and staff are specifically and deliberately assembled to help craft organizational direction and strategy, the healthcare team is more likely to support and "own" those change efforts. Having physicians side-by-side with administrative leadership is an inclusive gesture of partnership that will foster collaboration to create a shared vision. A vision should be a homegrown, easy-to-convey message that will resonate with every member of the healthcare team and the community it serves. It will, in essence, become the organization's "brand," marketplace differentiator, marketing pathway, signature, and what the system becomes known for. The values and principles of an organization's vision should be used for staff and physician selection, orientation, training, and systemwide behavioral standards. The vision should be widely projected, highly visible, and thoroughly understood by every member of the team, and held proudly at the center of the entire enterprise.

The following is an example of an organizational vision:

"Our commitment to our patients is to provide the best, most advanced healthcare that medical science has to offer and to treat our patients like they were members of our own family. We will listen, do the things we say we will do, explain every part of care, answer questions in a kind, caring spirit, and work as a team with patients to achieve the best outcome."

A clear and effective vision provides a strong sense of organizational character with extensive reach and significant influence on staff and physician behaviors. An organizational vision should span every level of the organization and be embraced, supported, and projected by every leader. The organizational vision should never be sequestered in a boardroom or strategy meeting, but serve as the pulse and fuel of all actions across the system.

2. **Communicate the vision to physicians.** Physician response to change is never good if they are caught by surprise. Use repetitive, deliberate communication with the medical staff to affirm that a renewed commitment to quality, service, and outcomes is coming. Communicating upcoming organizational strategies so there is clarity and understanding will lay the foundation for moving and changing together. Physicians who are unaware of proposed changes are far more likely to resist.

3. **Embrace a repetitive, multi-channel approach to physician communication.** There is no singular method of leader communication where every affiliated and employed medical staff member will hear and understand what is happening. I

frequently hear leaders say, "We told our physicians what was happening in an e-mail." That is not sufficient. Physician knowledge of vision and goals is a prerequisite for their support. Leadership communication must come in multiple formats and be repeated over time to assure that physicians hear it.

Multi-channel communication to physicians includes:

a. **Rounding on physicians.** In order to gain physician support and alignment for change efforts, leaders must spend time with physicians. Leaders cannot engage their medical staff from an office. Rounding on physicians is a strategy to build relationships and establish sincere two-way communication between administrative leadership and the medical staff. Leaders must spend time where physicians congregate, communicating change efforts and getting physician input regarding organizational intentions. The importance and value of leader visibility cannot be overstated. Spending time, face-to-face, is how the foundation of physician partnership is built.

b. **Newsletters.** Newsletters explaining the organizational commitment, goals, action plans, and timeline should be printed on brightly colored paper and placed in the physician lounge. They help communicate that a renewed, outcomes-driven focus is underway.

c. **E-mails.** Set up a regular e-mail communication from the executive team to physicians regarding upcoming initiatives. The most effective e-mail communication is the one that comes directly from the CEO. Send monthly updates regarding activities that support the new organizational vision and direction.

d. **Video streamed to the physician lounge.** Spending time with physicians is the most effective communication strategy. To reinforce the content of leader rounding, create a 15-

minute summary review of vision, goals, and strategies. Include your physician leadership and create a compelling summary of future aspirations. Play the video in the physician lounge or other places where physicians congregate. A video link can also be sent to the medical staff e-mail list to ensure the message is projected to the entire medical staff.

e. **CEO phone calls.** Face time with medical staff members can be a challenge, even for dedicated leadership. The scheduling of CEO phone calls to selected members of the medical staff is a powerful strategy to communicate and share information and to get physician input. Calls can be scheduled in 10-15-minute spots to share upcoming activities and to truly partner one-on-one with physicians. A personal phone call from the CEO asking for support and sharing organizational intentions is a powerful step toward creating the sense that this effort is different, and that the partnership is genuine.

f. **CEO letters.** Letters written to medical staff members from the CEO, addressed personally, signed, and sent to a physician's home are likely to be read. A clear, compelling vision of hospital and physician collaboration dedicated to superior outcomes and extraordinary service in the spirit of physician partnership can create understanding that something new is coming.

g. **Meet and greet.** The executive team can personally invite 10-15 physicians for an evening wine and cheese social gathering. Physicians will have a chance to get to know each other and members of the executive team in a less formal setting. Leaders will have an opportunity to get physician input, communicate upcoming activities, and build a true partnership of working together where both physicians and the system "win."

The effectiveness of leadership communication with physicians can determine the fate of the organizational vision. Leaders must "own" this effort. Leaders will need to generate and inspire enthusiasm in others that something different is underway. Passion, intensity, courage, and commitment must be projected by the leadership team. If communication of vision and goals is done with a sense of indifference, change efforts can stall before they begin. Key physicians in which strong relationships exist should be targeted for their leadership and support. Leaders will need the voice and support of key physicians early in this communication effort. This effort should never be perceived as an administrative activity, but rather a collaborative partnership moving together with physician leader visibility and support.

The communication of an organizational vision and strategy can take several months, but will speed downstream implementation efforts by reducing protest and creating physician support proactively. The investment of time and resources to communicate the direction, commitment, and vision of the organization to physicians is the initial step to effectively initiate the physician engagement process. When physicians know exactly what is coming and have been asked for genuine input early on, consensus and unity can be created. When consensus is achieved, the foundation for physician partnership is set.

ORGANIZATIONS THAT ALREADY HAVE A "VISION"

Many organizations will already have a preexisting vision. Leaders must ask themselves whether this vision is clear, well understood, and embraced across the organization, or whether it is burrowed in the halls of the facility with marginal awareness and influence.

If an organizational vision has faded with little impact on daily operations, the vision can be modified and refreshed to do what it is intended to do. The revision of an organizational direction can occur during the annual strategic planning that cycles in every organization. A renewed focus and vision is often what is needed to provide clarity to a fresh organizational effort. During the planning session, the physician communication and involvement strategies can be engaged as articulated in this stage. Deliberate, genuine, and early inclusion of the medical staff must be a part of any renewed commitment to substantive organizational change.

USING THE ORGANIZATIONAL VISION AS A MARKETING PLATFORM

Early in the Sharp HealthCare journey, I would see our commercials for our own system being projected over prime-time airways conveying our commitment to patients. It was very compelling to see what our patients were seeing. Our own marketing campaign created an effective internal "burning platform" to actually do what we said we would. Our commercials communicated our vision to our marketplace, but equally important, to ourselves. As I saw patients, I knew they had seen these commercials and felt I had to deliver on the commitment we had made to them. Our physicians felt that we could never be a party to a system that said one thing and did another. When I did my first training for our medical staff, I started the session by playing our commercials and everyone began to understand where we needed to go.

By projecting our commitment throughout the community, affiliated physicians, who are inherently more challenging to reach, saw our successfully executed marketing campaign. Though our marketing campaign was intended for patients, it also served as a powerful outreach to physicians to convey the spirit and vision of the Sharp Experience.

Repetitive, "multi-channel" communication, supported and projected by a marketing campaign, will promote physicians' understanding of and provide visibility for organizational efforts.

When a vision is developed, endorsed, communicated, and then advertised, an organization will have just created a powerful and visible platform to fully embed its own systemwide commitment. The impact of an organizational vision on physicians and every healthcare team member will be greater when a visible pledge to the marketplace has been made. A strong vision statement, visible in and out of the organization is, in and of itself, a change driver. A compelling vision that is communicated to patients creates commitment and accountability to walk the talk. A highly visible and well-projected vision conveys that there is no turning back and this IS what the organization will become. The reputation and credibility of the entire institution are at stake to execute the vision and deliver on the pledge.

SELECT ORGANIZATIONAL GOALS IN SUPPORT OF THE VISION

Though the vision of the organization will convey system intentions and identity, organizational performance is ultimately about the *execution* of goals. Vision without goals is soft and will not engage physicians. Conversely, goals without vision will fail to unify the healthcare workforce in a common, worthy effort to achieve transformational change.

In order to engage and partner with physicians to execute a vision, the vision and goals must be based on sound logic, physician input, and medical evidence. When goals are selected using these criteria and clearly linked to a well-understood, communicated, and supported vision, the foundation is set to establish a *shared* physician/system agenda. Setting goals is an endeavor pursued by most systems. The deliberate inclusion of physicians in goal selection is done less frequently.

The goals of the system must align with what is important to physicians in order for physicians to be vested in and committed to achieving these goals. When hospital leaders present *their* goals and *their* agenda on *their* terms, physicians will often respond with indifference and apathy. Physicians care about what impacts physicians and patients, and organizational goals must be crafted and communicated with this in mind. Physicians care about clinical quality, practice efficiency, the quality and training of the nurses they work with, profitability, their reputation among patients, staff, and colleagues, their input on issues, appreciation for what they do, and responsiveness to practice concerns. Leadership communication of vision and goals to physicians must be done with awareness and appreciation of what is important to physicians.

At Studer Group, we guide systems to create goals under Pillars of Performance to assure that every component of organizational performance is addressed. System goals should be balanced to create clear and measurable objectives representing clinical, operational, financial, and service performance, positioned and communicated in terms that will resonate with the medical staff.

System Performance Pillars include:

I. QUALITY PILLAR: Reflects quality processes and outcomes to measure and report clinical performance.

II. SERVICE PILLAR: Reflects the patient experience within the system. Goals in the service pillar reflect patient satisfaction and loyalty.

III. PEOPLE PILLAR: Reflects the workforce experience including physician and employee satisfaction.

IV. FINANCE PILLAR: Reflects financial performance including revenue, expenses, margins, and costs.

V. GROWTH PILLAR: Reflects system growth and market share.

Creating organizational pillar goals serves a number of important functions for system change and physician engagement. First, it provides clarity of objectives that are easily communicated. Conveyance of a system strategy to physicians must be efficient, well-organized, and communicated as goals that are relevant to them. Second, a pillar-based organizational strategy transitions physician perception of change efforts from a soft organizational vision to an evidence-based performance culture with clear outcome measures. Establishing and communicating goals that align with what physicians believe is important is a precursor and requirement for effective physician engagement. Specific goals across pillars for hospital, clinic, and emergency room environments will be reviewed in Stage 6, "Physician Measurement and Balanced Scorecards."

GETTING PHYSICIANS TO SUPPORT GOALS

Developing and communicating an organizational vision to physicians in the absence of system goals is likely to be seen as a fleeting effort with little substance or credibility. Leader communication to physicians should leave them fully informed of the scope of any change effort, and respectful of the depth of the organization's commitment to improve. In order to create the physician perception of an outcomes-based organization, physicians must not only understand the vision, strategy, and goals, but they must philosophically support the goals as important and attainable.

Tactics to create physician support for organizational goals:

a. **Physician leadership needs to be at the table to have a voice and input on system goal selection.** Physician leaders are far more likely to generate physician colleague support for performance goals if they were responsible for their selection.

b. **Goals should be based on compelling logic and evidence.** Every goal selected must have a specific return on investment or outcome benefit for the system, staff, physicians, or patients. Leaders must be able to "defend" goals based on a well-thought-out, evidence-based selection strategy. The certainty of the "why" of each goal will predict physician receptiveness to goal pursuit.

   The "why" might be evidence that implementing order sets for management of ventilated patients reduces ventilatory-associated pneumonias, or that patients given standardized post-operative thrombo-embolic prophylaxis have fewer embolic events. Sometimes, the "why" can be a story of a patient harmed by a renegade physician who refuses to adopt evidence-derived care pathways. A compelling "why" and supporting data reduce physician resistance and justify tactics to execute a goal.

c. **Goals selected must have leader consensus support.** If physician leaders fail to promote and support organizational goals or strategies to physician colleagues, rollout of goals to the general medical staff is going to be difficult, if not impossible. The leadership team must secure consensus on goals and strategy prior to taking action to achieve goals. Administrative and physician leadership must agree on what the system will pursue. The influence of the leadership voice on physicians' perceptions of vision and goals will be related to the *unity* of the message coming from the leadership team. A fractured and disconnected leadership message will make medical staff buy-in far more challenging.

Physicians are more likely to walk down a path whose coordinates are clear, logical, based on evidence, and convincingly communicated by high-performing leaders they respect. The details of the vision must be compelling, refreshing, and even inspiring to generate medical staff interest, support, and "buzz" for a system effort.

Initial communication efforts are important as they will determine the "first impression" many physicians will have regarding new strategies. Physicians will embrace well-prepared, effective leadership efforts that are logical and worthy. However, they will be relatively unforgiving of timid, administrative activities that are not well-organized and ineffectively communicated.

The following leader communication guidelines help ensure that physicians have a positive initial impression of the organizational vision and goals:

1. **Take time.** Use "multi-channel" communications to repeatedly, consistently, and deliberately project vision, goals, and strategy from executive leaders in a uniform voice. Communication of the organizational mission can take several months for all of the medical staff to hear and understand it. Physician awareness and support of change strategies must be in place *prior* to implementing action plans to achieve goals.

2. **Physician and administrative leadership teams should share the stage.** This organizational effort should never be portrayed or communicated as a hospital-based administrative agenda. When executive leaders are communicating change efforts and a renewed organizational vision, they should do so with physician

leaders at their side. Physician leaders need to be associated and visible in the initial communications with the general medical staff. Leader unity is key to diminish the "we/they" attitude that can undermine change efforts. Physician leadership linkage and association with the vision and strategy will motivate physician leaders to "sell" the message to the general medical staff more effectively.

3. **Present changes as a win-win strategy.** Physicians are trained to be critical and are likely to be suspicious of initial organizational change efforts. To offset suspicion, leaders must communicate organizational strategies in the genuine spirit of "win-win." If leaders are unable to clearly communicate how an organizational effort will benefit physicians, then the strategy should be redesigned. Physicians will listen to leaders and embrace strategies if they believe that doing so will benefit them in meaningful ways. Physician benefits may include:
   - Financial incentives for quality and service performance (employed model)
   - Improved OR start times
   - Improved nursing communication to physicians
   - Improved follow-up care through discharge phone calls
   - Increased efficiency in the clinical care of patients
   - Greater physician input into quality and operational issues
   - Improved physician satisfaction as an organizational goal
   - Renewed leadership focus to meet the needs of the medical staff
   - Improved communication between leadership and physicians

Communicate the organizational vision in terms that are meaningful for physicians to garner their support. Make the renewed organizational direction and proposed future of the institution "irresistible" to the medical staff.

4. **Make the case for Why.** Medicare reform, pay-for-performance, public transparency, rising competition for favorable payers, nonreimbursable Never Events, nursing pool shortages, diminishing revenues, and Joint Commission regulations are progressive environmental conditions that mandate healthcare system performance and efficiency. Leaders will need to present a rock-solid case to physicians much like an attorney makes a case in a courtroom. System change can be challenging, but the consequences for failing to respond to current conditions can be far worse. Leaders should not be timid or hesitant. The message needs to be logical and based on industry evidence. The vision and goals articulated in Stage 1 are a means to improve quality outcomes, build patient loyalty, improve financial performance, improve physician satisfaction, reduce staff turnover, improve employee satisfaction, reduce malpractice risk, and improve the care experience for physicians, staff, and employees. The likelihood of physician "rejection" or indifference toward vision and goals is diminished when physicians understand why changes *must* be made.

5. **Communicate organizational objectives in physician-centric terms.** To be frank, physicians may not care about a hospital's commitment to the "new agenda." If this effort is positioned and communicated simply as a hospital-driven agenda, leaders may watch a room full of physicians collectively play with their BlackBerries. The KEY to communication is to create common goals that matter to physicians. These goals can be divided into the strategic pillars serving global performance objectives. Position the renewed organizational commitments as "evidence-based and outcomes-driven." We describe our work at Studer Group in these terms and it aligns well with how physicians think. Pillar objectives communicated in physician-centric terms include the following:

A. **Quality**-Hospital leaders care about CMS core measure performance; physicians care about evidence-based medicine to create improved outcomes for patients. Place system goals in the *physicians'* terms, not the hospital's. Core measures are frequently measurements of processes, and can sound sterile and "regulatory." When communicating quality aspirations, clinical processes must be profiled as links to improved patient outcomes when speaking of a quality commitment to physicians. "Saving lives" and "improved outcomes" speaks to physicians: "CMS core measures" is less appealing. Linking processes to clinical outcomes is a more compelling communication style with physicians. This communication to physicians can include:

1. Acute Myocardial Infarction Measures:
   - Patients given an aspirin upon arrival at the hospital have a 23 percent less chance of dying within the next 35 days.
   - Patients who continue to take aspirin after leaving the hospital have a 23 percent less chance of having another heart problem or heart-related death.
   - Patients given a beta-blocker upon arrival have a 14 percent less chance of dying within one week.
   - Patients prescribed a beta-blocker when leaving the hospital have a 28 percent less chance of having another myocardial infarction.

2. CHF Measures:
   - Patients prescribed an ACE inhibitor have a 20 percent less chance of dying within one year.

3. Pneumonia Measures:
    - Patients who get a pneumonia vaccination before leaving the hospital have a 43 percent less chance of being hospitalized and a 29 percent less chance of dying from pneumonia.[1]

B. **Efficiency**-Physicians will often rate the "quality" of a hospital by the efficiency of their practice experience and not necessarily by the hospital's clinical performance. Efficiency and improving the physician work experience should be at the forefront of the communication of the organizational commitment to physicians. The leadership message to physicians should be: *Our goal is to eliminate barriers to care and to eliminate those things that waste your time.* System efficiency and organizational responsiveness to physicians' concerns will ultimately determine the judgment a physician passes on a system, its leadership team, and the renewed commitment to change.

C. **People**-People pillar objectives are performance commitments related to the workforce, including physicians, nurses, and ancillary personnel. They include measures of employee satisfaction, physician satisfaction, and turnover. Physicians need to hear that leadership is committed to becoming the employer of choice, with a clinical environment built on collaboration, respect, teamwork, and performance. Physicians want to be treated well, but they also need to see a commitment to high-quality staff and the highest priority placed on the system's human resources. People pillar goals of employee and physician satisfaction as a communicated system commitment will improve physicians' perception of the organization and its goals.

D. **Service**-When a patient's likelihood of recommending a hospital increases, so does the physician's loyalty to the hospital.[2] Satisfied patients make for satisfied employees and physicians, and satisfied employees and physicians will provide better care to patients. Physicians prefer to affiliate with organizations that provide exceptional care to their patients. Rounding on patients who complain to physicians about the service and care they receive makes for an aggravating physician experience and can be enough to take their patients elsewhere. As leaders communicate the vision and strategy of the organization, the patient experience should be at the center of efforts. A word of advice: When communicating service goals to the medical staff, do not stand in front of a roomful of physicians and speak of increasing "patient satisfaction scores." Physicians do not really care about "scores," but they care a great deal about providing quality care, improving the patient experience, and strengthening their reputation and the reputation of the facility where they work. Patient experience and service goals align closely with a physician's personal desire to be successful. An organizational ambition to provide exceptional service to patients is a simple and clear collaborative opportunity to create a shared direction with physicians. Creating a mutually beneficial agenda with physicians is a core element of the physician engagement process.

6. **Articulate the physician role.** Physicians are frequently willing to partner to achieve worthy goals, but they often don't know what is expected of them. It is important to clearly communicate the physician role in the organizational mission early. Elements of the physician role include:

A. *How physicians treat patients:* A principal predictor of the patient experience in the clinic and hospital environment is how physicians interact and communicate with patients. As a system that will be built and differentiated by the patient experience, clarity and consistency of physician conduct is key.

B. *How physicians treat staff:* A driver and predictor of clinical safety, staff retention, and employee satisfaction is how physicians communicate with nurses. The culture and reputation of a system will hinge on physicians' conduct toward staff, and this will serve as a critical component to the physician role in organizational efforts.

C. *How physicians treat colleagues:* The quality of relationships and interactions that physicians have with each other will influence a physician's clinical and personal experience within a system. The physician role in creating a collaborative, collegial, and friendly clinical environment among fellow medical staff members should be a clearly communicated physician responsibility in a system committed to safety, quality, and service.

Leadership communication with physicians should place them in a position of impact as the clinical workplace leaders. Leaders should reach out to physicians as a gesture of partnership and communicate that full achievement of common goals can happen only with the active leadership and example set by physicians. Leaders should express the sentiment, *We cannot do this without our physicians.* Physicians inherently appreciate being positioned as the clinical leader and having influence, and they will frequently embrace the responsibility and opportunity of making others better.

SUMMARY

Creating and communicating a bold and compelling organizational vision in partnership with physicians is the first stage of the physician engagement sequence. Failure to create and lead an organization that is driven by a common vision will make partnership, collaboration, and coordination of efforts far more challenging. Getting a system to work together requires unity and a common, shared purpose to carry out the mission.

Unified systems can withstand resistance, press through, stay together, look out for each other, and help one another to make a difference and achieve something extraordinary.

A clear, logical, articulated roadmap to achieve pillar-based results, with goals that matter to physicians, lays the foundation for partnership in a new, shared agenda. Do not be afraid of ambition, passion, and enthusiasm when communicating with physicians. Physicians want the same things as other healthcare team members, and will gravitate to visionary leaders who are willing to step up and drive outcomes. The creation and communication of a collaborative vision and common goals will launch the journey of *Engaging Physicians.*

Key Learnings for Stage 1, "Create and Communicate Organizational Vision and Goals":

1. Assemble physician leaders, select physicians, nursing team members, and administrative leadership together to create (or renew) an organizational vision.
2. The vision should be simple, easy to convey, and representative of what the organization "aspires to be."
3. Consider using the organizational vision as a marketing signature to bring a message to the marketplace and to widely project change efforts inside and outside of the organization.
4. Create a balanced set of goals across pillars that represent the "execution" of the vision. Physician leadership should be involved and have input into goal selection.
5. Organizational goals should:
    a. Be based on medical evidence
    b. Generate specific return on investment for the system
    c. Generate benefits for patients, physicians, or staff
6. Communicate vision and goals to medical staff from physician leadership, standing together with administrative leadership as a unified voice. Communication should be well-organized with a clear strategy and defined outcomes across pillars.
7. Use "physician-centric" language when communicating system goals to physicians.
8. Communicate organizational vision, strategy, and goals repeatedly using a "multi-channel" approach to ensure reaching the medical staff. Rounding on physicians and personal leader contact are the most effective strategies for communicating the message.

STAGE 2:
Leadership Development and Accountability for Performance

"Vision without execution is hallucination."
—Thomas Edison

In order for physicians to engage in a system effort, those leading the effort must have credibility and earn the respect of physicians. Leader credibility in the eyes of physicians is about leaders improving outcomes, driving change, and effectively delivering on the stated vision of the organization. Ineffective leaders who struggle to create consensus, who fail to inspire others, who stumble when challenged, and seem unable to lead meaningful change will have a hard time convincing physicians to join their teams. Physicians are watching, and the credibility of the leadership team weighs in the balance. The level of leader credibility will heavily influence the effectiveness and thoroughness of the physician engagement effort.

For leaders to execute outcomes and effectively build credibility, several critical organizational activities must occur. These include:

1. **Setting clear organizational goals (Stage 1)**
2. **Developing the leadership team and providing leaders with skills to drive outcomes**
3. **Developing an individual leader evaluation process that assesses a leader's performance by an ability to achieve specific performance goals**

Stage 2, "Leadership Development and Accountability for Performance," is a pathway to a leadership-driven outcomes culture that will serve as the engine for organizational change. Effective leadership is a requisite for physician engagement, as physicians are quick to pass judgment on ineffective change efforts. Leadership Development and Accountability for Performance is a tested leadership model that delivers measurable results across pillars. Measurable and significant leader results will help avoid early dismissal of organizational strategies from a frequently skeptical and cynical medical staff.

From a physician's perspective, the commitment to a renewed vision articulated in Stage 1 is still just leaders' words awaiting action. Vision and goals without action and results will fade quickly in the eyes of an observant medical staff. The progress and momentum of physician engagement will ultimately depend on leaders' demonstrating an ability to implement strategies to *execute* the vision. If goals and vision are communicated and not manifested, then this will just be "another example" of administration not doing what they said they would.

Joint Commissions Executive Quality Improvement Survey, published in the *Journal of Patient Safety* in March 2006, reported that, "Leadership has been identified as the most important ingredient in transformational improvement." Leader performance is a core element of physician partnership and a uniform feature of systems that earn the respect, confidence, and esteem of physicians. Physicians are far more likely to align with effective leaders who enroll others in a systemwide change and take visible action to achieve a worthy vision.

Though leader performance is clearly an important precursor to the physician engagement process, the effectiveness of leaders will ultimately determine nearly all organizational performance outcomes. Leadership Development and Accountability for Performance are key elements to position system leaders to achieve results and are central properties of high-performing organizations.

When Studer Group coaches healthcare systems, creating balanced pillar-based goals, developing effective leaders, and implementing an objective evaluation system for individual leader performance are foundational strategies for organizational improvement. Why is individual accountability so important? First, it clearly connects the goals of the organization to the individual leader. Second, accountability allows senior leaders to continuously monitor leader performance. Third, leader evaluation based on objective pillar goals keeps leaders focused on what's important and intensifies a leader's effort to achieve outcomes.

When a system CEO stands in front of a group of managers and articulates a solid "system plan" to increase quality and service as an organizational commitment, improved performance in quality and service may or may not happen. Conversely, if this CEO were to cascade those quality and service goals down to individual managers and hold them accountable for service and quality results on their units, performance improvement becomes more likely.

In his book *Hardwiring Excellence* Quint Studer writes, "If there are only a few things you do, let one be the adoption of an objective measurable leader evaluation tool. Then hold leaders accountable for those results."

LEADERSHIP DEVELOPMENT

Many leaders within healthcare systems, particularly physicians, have little training to lead. Leadership development will focus on key leader competencies to achieve outcomes. Running effective meetings, managing financial resources, answering tough questions so as to not create a "we/they" culture, selecting talent, having difficult conversations with low performers, and understanding the external environment are trainable leader skills that will improve leader performance.

At Studer Group, our partners provide "Leadership Development Institutes" (LDIs) for leaders, including physician leaders, on a quarterly basis to ensure that key skills are in place at every level. The benefits of leadership development include the abilities to customize training to the organization's needs, to build team member relationships across the system through networking, and to integrate physician and administrative leadership to develop common skills simultaneously.

Over the years, with hundreds of partner organizations, we have seen a broad spectrum of LDIs. Most are successful in implementing strategies and developing leader skills to create outcomes. Some LDIs are less successful in creating leader change and system results. When organizational leaders fail to create results, training philosophies can sometimes descend into a culture of "rationalization" for poor performance and "optionalization" for member participation. If leaders cloak LDIs with rationalization and optionalization, attendees will walk away with little pressure to change what they do. Great leaders must drive training, make no excuses for performance, and expect everyone across the system to be enrolled in the effort. LDIs are the forum where leaders can project current performance, initiate strategies, and convey a relentless organizational will to get the work done.

The argument and evidence for investing in leaders is replicated in many industries. *BusinessWeek* in October 2005 reported, "Companies who invest in leadership development outperform the competition." *BusinessWeek* also reports, "Among employees who say their company offers poor development opportunities, 41 percent plan to leave within 12 months versus only 12 percent who rate their opportunities as excellent." Former CEO of Pepsi Steve Reinemund said it best, "If the people don't grow, the company doesn't grow."

Physician leaders should attend LDI sessions. Physician leaders who do not participate in leadership development risk dividing an organization along the lines of physicians and administration. This two-part structure moves slower, encounters more resistance, hears more protest, and will be challenged to transform itself. Conversely, physician leader presence as a voice of leadership in support of change efforts creates an important sense of organizational unity. Administrative leadership becomes more effective when they are supported and backed by visible, engaged, and participatory physician leaders.

Specific content and topics for LDIs are available within our website at www.studergroup.com. Examples of LDI topics can include the following:

1. **Service Training**-How to train others in the delivery of service excellence
2. **"Rounding for Outcomes"**-How to use rounding on leaders/direct report/employees/physicians and patients to drive results
3. **Difficult Conversations**-How to have critical communications with low performers
4. **A Culture of Safety**-How to create a "speak-up" organization
5. **Behavioral Standards**-How to create and implement a Code of Conduct that changes employee/physician behavior

6. **Employee/Physician Selection**-How to use behavioral interviewing to find a cultural match with employees and physician hires
7. **Engaging the Workforce**-How to create focus and alignment of the entire organization to achieve a renewed vision
8. **Improving Employee Satisfaction**-How to reduce turnover and improve employee satisfaction

Leadership Development Institutes are places to build teams, develop tactics, and learn what message needs to cascade to the rest of the workforce. Attendance is a privilege and comes with the expectation that attendees deliver on plans of action.

LEADERSHIP ACCOUNTABILITY

When individual leaders are assessed not on "attitude" or projects, but on measurable results, a leader's focus and effort to achieve goals intensifies. *Results* are the measure of effective leadership, and organizational leader evaluation methods must reflect this.

Accountability is about holding leaders responsible for getting things done. In the end, outcomes are what matter, and *results* are what make organizations great. In the absence of accountability, the reliability of leader performance is compromised. It is vision and strategy that guide organizations, and leadership development that grows a skilled leadership team, but it is leader accountability that drives outcomes. Individual accountability has a heavy influence on human behaviors and underlies much of a workforce's efforts.

We all have personal encounters with the impact of accountability, and the fundamental effect it has on what we do. I have lived in our neighborhood for the last eight years with a busy four-way traffic light that I pass through going to and from work every day. For many years, when the light turned yellow, I would do as I always did, which was to step firmly on the accelerator to get through the intersection before the light turned red. While driving home one early evening, the light turned yellow, and I stepped firmly on the gas pedal. A subtle but distinct flash appeared as I sped through the intersection. One week later, I was sent a photo of myself with a moving violation citation and a fine for over $350. Apparently, this camera was installed because of people like me. I still pass the intersection every day, but now press on the brake when the light turns yellow. Every time. Consistent behavioral change in the absence of accountability can be as probable as me slowing for the yellow light without a traffic camera.

Martin Luther King once said, "Leaders begin to lead when they see the light, or feel the heat." System vision and leader development are about helping leaders to become inspired and "see the light," and to be a part of a team that is dedicated to making a difference and creating a workplace that is unified to make the lives of patients better. Inspiration is important and necessary to make an organization great, but inspiration alone, without accountability, will not assure a culture of execution. Embedding accountability will guide a vision-driven organization to continually improve. Building accountability is about clarifying expectations, verifying individual performance, and creating a method to cascade organizational pillar goals down to individual leaders.

How does individual leader accountability work? Every leader, from the CEO and the executive team to individual physician leaders down to unit managers, should have a specified "goal set" across pillars. In order for leaders to achieve goals, specific expectations of individual performance must be made clear. Each goal used to evaluate leader performance should be objective and measurable for quality, service, people, growth and finance that are specific for individual leaders. Leaders are assigned only goals that are within their scope of influence and responsibility and relate specifically to the performance of their led "unit." The CFO is unlikely to have clinical marker performance on his/her goals, and the CMO is unlikely to have bed turnover times and nurse turnover rates.

Accountability and visibility of individual leader performance can and will create tension in an organization. The days of leaders "getting by" and "faking it" are done. An objective leader evaluation system will provide clarity, and a sometimes brutal reality, of leader performance.

When I have spoken to medical staff leadership about holding physician leaders accountable for results, the room will typically fall silent for a few moments. Recently in one of these training sessions, a physician leader broke the silence and said, "So *I* am going to be held responsible for CMS core measure performance?" He wondered how in the world he *alone* could drive the entire system to achieve top decile core measure performance. I informed him that in an era of leader accountability, his leadership would be assessed by his results, including system core measure performance. I assured him that many excellent leaders in clinical positions would have core measures on their goal set, and they too would be intensely focused on getting things done. He felt better, and saw the logic of accountability and transparency of performance as a way of focusing leader actions to a collective and unified effort.

Every leader is assigned goals that "match" the organizational goals, but are customized and weighted according to a leader's position, responsibilities, and the specific unit that he or she leads or manages.

As an example, a nurse manager of a surgical unit may have a "goal set" across pillars that can look something like this:

SERVICE: Improve patient satisfaction to the 80th percentile in the surgical unit, with a stretch goal of the 85th percentile. Current performance is the 70th percentile.

PEOPLE: Reduce nurse turnover to 16 percent, with a stretch goal of 14 percent. Current performance is 18 percent turnover.

FINANCE: Improve unit patient discharge times to 80 percent discharges completed by noon on the surgical unit, with a stretch goal of 85 percent. Current performance is 54 percent.

QUALITY: Goal 1) Reduce fall rates by 30 percent with a stretch goal of 40 percent.

Goal 2) Reduce hospital-acquired decubiti by 30 percent with a stretch goal of 40 percent.

GROWTH: Reduce average length of stay on the surgical unit to 3.65 with a stretch goal of 3.57. Current performance is 3.80.

Leaders are given a "score" on a 5-point scale based on their performance across individual pillar goals. Typically, a "4" is given for hitting a goal, and a "5" for hitting a stretch goal, though the rating scale can be adjusted. Assessment, reporting, and visibility of performance of the stated "goal set" give an objective report of who is getting what done. Ideally, this dashboard of individual leader performance is one that is web-based, auto uploads, and is visible from anywhere with all individual leader evaluations assembled in a centralized, easy-to-navigate location. The ideal leader evaluation tool should have the ability to "weight" quality, service, growth, and financial goals and create unique goal sets that are specified to individual leader roles. This web-based leader scorecard is developed and deployed as the Studer Group software system, "Leadership Evaluation Manager" (LEM). LEM is used by many of our partners and healthcare systems across the country to assist executive teams with individual leader accountability and real-time leader performance assessment.

The following is an example of a hospital CEO goal set presented on the Leader Evaluation Manager software program:

Figure 2.1

LEADER EVALUATION MANAGER - CEO SAMPLE

Pillar	Goals							
			1	2	3	4	5	
Service Weighted Value 20%	**Goal:** Increase patient satisfaction to the 75th percentile in IP, OP, and ED **Result:** 56 for Jan thru Dec *» add goal* *» remove this goal*	» Edit Rating Type Percentile **Higher is better** **5** is 85 and above **4** is 75 to 84 **3** is 65 to 74 **2** is 55 to 64 **1** is 54 and below	20% v Weighted Value	x	2 Score	=	0.4 Item Score	
			1	2	3	4	5	
Quality Weighted Value 15%	**Goal:** Reduce patient fall rate to 0.1 fall per 1,000 patient days. **Result:** 0.161 for Jan thru Dec *» add goal* *» remove this goal*	» Edit Rating Type Falls per 1,000 PDs **Lower is better** **5** is .05 and below **4** is .075 to 0.051 **3** is .1 to 0.076 **2** is .15 to 0.101 **1** is 0.151 and above	15% v Weighted Value	x	1 Score	=	0.15 Item Score	
			1	**2**	3	4	5	
People Weighted Value 15%	**Goal:** Reduce employee turnover to 12%. **Result:** 16 for Jan thru Dec *» add goal* *» remove this goal*	» Edit Rating Type Turnover % **Lower is better** **5** is 10.4 and below **4** is 12 to 10.5 **3** is 14 to 12.1 **2** is 16 to 14.1 **1** is 16.1 and above	15% v Weighted Value	x	2 Score	=	0.3 Item Score	
			1	**2**	3	4	5	
Finance Weighted Value 35%	**Goal:** Increase operating margin to 3% **Result:** 2.1 for Jan thru Dec *» add goal* *» remove this goal*	» Edit Rating Type % **Higher is better** **5** is 3.5 and above **4** is 3.0 to 3.4 **3** is 2.5 to 2.9 **2** is 2 to 2.4 **1** is 1.9 and below	25% v Weighted Value	x	2 Score	=	0.5 Item Score	

Pillar	Goals							
Finance (con't) Weighted Value 35%	**Goal:** Increase days cash on hand to 120. **Result:** 112 for Jan thru Dec » *add goal* » *remove this goal*	» Edit Rating Type Days Cash on Hand **Higher is better** **5** is 130 and above **4** is 120 to 129 **3** is 110 to 119 **2** is 100 to 109 **1** is 99 and below	1 10% Weighted Value	2 x	**3** 3 Score	4 =	5 0.3 Item Score	
Growth Weighted Value 15%	**Goal:** Increase adjusted admissions to 8,500. **Result:** 8,616 for Jan thru Dec » *add goal* » *remove this goal*	» Edit Rating Type Adjusted Admissions **Higher is better** **5** is 9,000 and above **4** is 8,500 to 8,999 **3** is 8,000 to 8,499 **2** is 7,500 to 7,999 **1** is 7,499 and below	1 15% Weighted Value	2 x	3 4 Score	**4** =	5 0.6 Item Score	
Total Weight: 100/100					**Overall Performance Score:** 2.25			

The LEM provides leaders an overall "score" based on the sum of individual pillar performance items between 1 and 5. The score is reflective of specific composite results across pillar goals. If a service goal represents 40 percent of a leader's evaluation, and that leader receives a "3" for service results on his or her unit, the item score for service will be .4 (40 percent) multiplied by "3" (score), which is equal to 1.2 item score under the service pillar goal. All pillars are calculated in a similar fashion to provide the overall leader score between 1 and 5. In the Studer Group user database, an average leader score is approximately 2.85. Scores greater than 4.45 are achieved by less than 5 percent of leaders.

The Leader Evaluation Manager or similar leader scorecard is the ultimate tool to assess, monitor, and verify individual performance across a system. Every leader's performance across his or her pillar-based "goal set" is visible on the web by any member of the leadership team. Leader scorecards serve as a sophisticated application of peer pressure, one of the most powerful drivers of human behavior. Visibility of performance through individual leader assessment will ensure that low performers feel pressure to improve, and that high performers receive the recognition they deserve.

The process of goal-setting, leadership development, and leadership accountability is referred to at Studer Group as "Evidence Based Leadership"℠ (EBL). Evidence Based Leadership is a tested and proven leadership model within the Studer Group partner data base to deliver superior outcomes across pillars compared to organizations that do not hold leaders accountable for performance. The summaries below are service results comparing organizations that have implemented individual leader accountability versus organizations that have not.

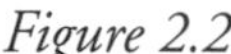

Figure 2.2

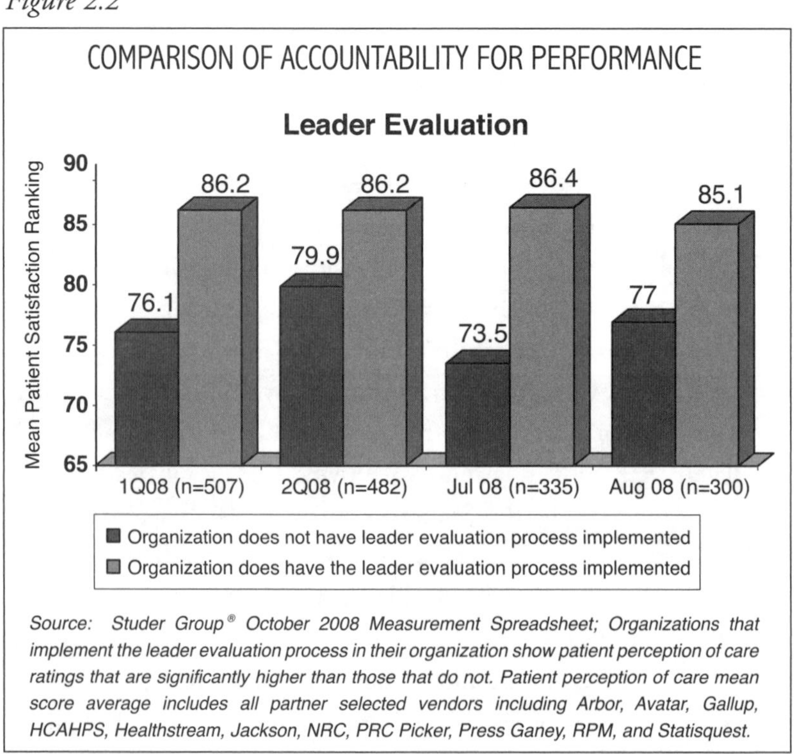

Source: Studer Group® October 2008 Measurement Spreadsheet; Organizations that implement the leader evaluation process in their organization show patient perception of care ratings that are significantly higher than those that do not. Patient perception of care mean score average includes all partner selected vendors including Arbor, Avatar, Gallup, HCAHPS, Healthstream, Jackson, NRC, PRC Picker, Press Ganey, RPM, and Statisquest.

Evidence Based Leadership is an accountability tool that should be shared and communicated to the general medical staff as a new way of running the organization. EBL is a shot across the bow to the medical staff that this initiative is of substance, change is real, and leaders are genuinely committed to delivering on an ambitious vision.

PHYSICIAN LEADER ACCOUNTABILITY FOR GOAL EXECUTION

Are physicians placed on this same leader evaluation system? In time, physician leaders who are employed can and should be placed on a leadership evaluation system.

Like any member of the system leadership team, physicians are also accountable for executing outcomes in support of system pillar goals. If physician leaders "voice support" for organizational efforts but resist personal accountability for performance, further physician alignment work needs to be done. If physician leaders are sincere in their support of a transformational journey, then accepting individual accountability to assure performance should not be protested. Great leaders are not dominated by personal agendas and individual accolades, but are driven by the pursuit of a higher and more important organizational mission.

The entry point for physician leaders embracing, or at least accepting, accountability for performance will depend on the system executive team leading the way. When the CEO stands in support of a new, bold, transformational vision and places his or her own scorecard in front of the entire physician leadership team, it can pave the way for physician leaders doing the same. The executive team can ask of physician leaders only what they have done themselves.

The content of a physician leader goal set will depend on the organization and its goals. The following is an example of a goal set for a Chief Medical Officer in an inpatient setting on the LEM software program:

Figure 2.3

LEADER EVALUATION MANAGER - INPATIENT PHYSICIAN LEADER SAMPLE

Pillar	Goals		
Service Weighted Value 25%	**Goal:** Improve patient satisfaction to the 80th percentile Current 76th percentile **Result:** 82 for Jan thru Dec *» add goal* *» remove this goal*	» Edit Rating Type Percentile **Higher is better** **5** is 90 and above **4** is 80 to 89 **3** is 70 to 79 **2** is 50 to 69 **1** is 49 and below	1 2 3 **4** 5 25% (Weighted Value) x 4 (Score) = 1 (Item Score)
Quality Weighted Value 40%	**Goal:** 95% of patients with LV dysfunction receive ACE/ARB at discharge **Result:** 84 for Jan thru Dec *» add goal* *» remove this goal*	» Edit Rating Type % **Higher is better** **5** is 97.6 and above **4** is 95 to 97.5 **3** is 92.5 to 94.9 **2** is 90 to 92.4 **1** is 89.9 and below	**1** 2 3 4 5 10% (Weighted Value) x 1 (Score) = 0.1 (Item Score)
	Goal: 94% of patients receive beta blocker at discharge for AMI **Result:** 91 for Jan thru Dec *» add goal* *» remove this goal*	» Edit Rating Type % **Higher is better** **5** is 97.1 and above **4** is 94 to 97 **3** is 91 to 93.9 **2** is 88 to 90.9 **1** is 87.9 and below	1 2 **3** 4 5 10% (Weighted Value) x 3 (Score) = 0.3 (Item Score)
	Goal: 90% of patients with CAP receive appropriate initial antibiotic **Result:** 92 for Jan thru Dec *» add goal* *» remove this goal*	» Edit Rating Type % **Higher is better** **5** is 96 and above **4** is 90 to 95 **3** is 86 to 89 **2** is 84 to 85 **1** is 83 and below	1 2 3 **4** 5 10% (Weighted Value) x 4 (Score) = 0.4 (Item Score)
	Goal: 98% of patients receive ASA at discharge for AMI **Result:** 94.5 for Jan thru Dec *» add goal* *» remove this goal*	» Edit Rating Type % **Higher is better** **5** is 98 and above **4** is 95 to 97.9 **3** is 92 to 94.9 **2** is 90 to 91.9 **1** is 89.9 and below	1 2 **3** 4 5 10% (Weighted Value) x 3 (Score) = 0.3 (Item Score)

Pillar	Goals	Rating Type	Rating Scale	Weighted Value		Score		Item Score
People Weighted Value 15%	**Goal:** Decrease employed physician turnover to 8.0% **Result:** 6.2 for Jan thru Dec » *add goal* » *remove this goal*	» Edit Rating Type % **Lower is better**	**5** is 6.5 and below **4** is 8 to 6.6 **3** is 10 to 8.1 **2** is 12 to 10.1 **1** is 12.1 and above	1 2 3 4 **5** 5% v Weighted Value	x	5 Score	=	0.25 Item Score
	Goal: Improve physician satisfaction to the 75th percentile **Result:** 54 for Jan thru Dec » *add goal* » *remove this goal*	» Edit Rating Type Percentile **Higher is better**	**5** is 80 and above **4** is 70 to 79 **3** is 60 to 69 **2** is 50 to 59 **1** is 49 and below	1 **2** 3 4 5 10% v Weighted Value	x	2 Score	=	0.2 Item Score
Finance Weighted Value 10%	**Goal:** Reduce acute Medicare LOS to 3.57 days or less **Result:** 3.78 for Jan thru Dec » *add goal* » *remove this goal*	» Edit Rating Type Days **Lower is better**	**5** is 3.57 and below **4** is 3.62 to 3.58 **3** is 3.66 to 3.63 **2** is 3.78 to 3.67 **1** is 3.79 and above	1 **2** 3 4 5 5% v Weighted Value	x	2 Score	=	0.1 Item Score
	Goal: Increase discharge order by noon to 90% **Result:** 68 for Jan thru Dec » *add goal* » *remove this goal*	» Edit Rating Type % **Higher is better**	**5** is 90 and above **4** is 80 to 89 **3** is 70 to 79 **2** is 60 to 69 **1** is 59 and below	1 **2** 3 4 5 5% v Weighted Value	x	2 Score	=	0.1 Item Score
Growth Weighted Value 10%	**Goal:** Improve likelihood to recommend hospital to 85th percentile **Result:** 84 for Jan thru Dec » *add goal* » *remove this goal*	» Edit Rating Type Percentile **Higher is better**	**5** is 90 and above **4** is 80 to 89 **3** is 70 to 79 **2** is 55 to 69 **1** is 54 and below	1 2 3 **4** 5 10% v Weighted Value	x	4 Score	=	0.4 Item Score
Total Weight: 100/100				**Overall Performance Score:** 3.15				

In this example, this physician leader's composite score is a 3.15 based on performance on an assigned goal set across pillars.

Here is an example of a goal set loaded on an LEM web-based system for an outpatient setting:

Figure 2.4

LEADER EVALUATION MANAGER - OUTPATIENT PHYSICIAN LEADER SAMPLE

Pillar	Goals							
Service Weighted Value 25%	**Goal:** Improve patient satisfaction to the 80th percentile **Result:** 58 for Jan thru Dec » *add goal* » *remove this goal*	» Edit Rating Type Percentile **Higher is better** **5** is 90 and above **4** is 80 to 89 **3** is 70 to 79 **2** is 50 to 69 **1** is 49 and below	1 / **2** / 3 / 4 / 5	25% Weighted Value	x	2 Score	=	0.5 Item Score
Quality Weighted Value 40%	**Goal:** 70% of patients with hypertension with BP <140/90 **Result:** 76 for Jan thru Dec » *add goal* » *remove this goal*	» Edit Rating Type % **Higher is better** **5** is 80 and above **4** is 70 to 79 **3** is 60 to 69 **2** is 50 to 59 **1** is 49 and below	1 / 2 / 3 / **4** / 5	10% Weighted Value	x	4 Score	=	0.4 Item Score
	Goal: 70% of patients with diabetes have an LDL <100 **Result:** 81 for Jan thru Dec » *add goal* » *remove this goal*	» Edit Rating Type % **Higher is better** **5** is 80 and above **4** is 70 to 79 **3** is 60 to 69 **2** is 50 to 59 **1** is 49 and below	1 / 2 / 3 / 4 / **5**	10% Weighted Value	x	5 Score	=	0.5 Item Score
	Goal: 7% of patients with DM hga1c >9.0 **Result:** 6.5 for Jan thru Dec » *add goal* » *remove this goal*	» Edit Rating Type % **Lower is better** **5** is 5 and below **4** is 7 to 5.1 **3** is 10 to 7.1 **2** is 13 to 10.1 **1** is 13.1 and above		10% Weighted Value	x	4 Score	=	0.4 Item Score

Pillar	Goals		
Quality (con't) Weighted Value 40%	**Goal:** 92% of women 40-70 with annual mammograms **Result:** 93 for Jan thru Dec » *add goal* » *remove this goal*	» Edit Rating Type % **Higher is better** **5** is 96 and above **4** is 92 to 95 **3** is 88 to 91 **2** is 84 to 87 **1** is 83 and below	1 2 3 **4** 5 10% Weighted Value × 4 Score = 0.4 Item Score
People Weighted Value 15%	**Goal:** Improve meeting attendance to 50% of staff meetings **Result:** 48 for Jan thru Dec » *add goal* » *remove this goal*	» Edit Rating Type % **Higher is better** **5** is 75 and above **4** is 50 to 74 **3** is 40 to 49 **2** is 30 to 39 **1** is 29 and below	1 2 **3** 4 5 5% Weighted Value × 3 Score = 0.15 Item Score
	Goal: Improve physician satisfaction by 10% compared to 2007 **Result:** 12 for Jan thru Dec » *add goal* » *remove this goal*	» Edit Rating Type % **Higher is better** **5** is 13 and above **4** is 10 to 12 **3** is 5 to 9 **2** is 0 to 4 **1** is -1 and below	1 2 3 **4** 5 10% Weighted Value × 4 Score = 0.4 Item Score
Finance Weighted Value 10%	**Goal:** Increase individual provider visits by 5% compared to 2007 **Result:** 2 for Jan thru Dec » *add goal* » *remove this goal*	» Edit Rating Type % **Higher is better** **5** is 7.5 and above **4** is 5 to 7.4 **3** is 2 to 4.9 **2** is 1 to 1.9 **1** is 0.9 and below	1 2 **3** 4 5 5% Weighted Value × 3 Score = 0.15 Item Score
	Goal: Improve generic medication use to 55% **Result:** 68 for Jan thru Dec » *add goal* » *remove this goal*	» Edit Rating Type % **Higher is better** **5** is 65 and above **4** is 55 to 64 **3** is 45 to 54 **2** is 35 to 44 **1** is 34 and below	1 2 3 4 **5** 5% Weighted Value × 5 Score = 0.25 Item Score

Pillar	Goals							
	Goal: Improve likelihood to recommend physicians to 85th percentile	» Edit Rating Type Percentile	1	**2**	3	4	5
Growth Weighted Value 10%	**Result:** 55 for Jan thru Dec » *add goal* » *remove this goal*	**Higher is better** **5** is 90 and above **4** is 80 to 89 **3** is 70 to 79 **2** is 55 to 69 **1** is 54 and below	10% Weighted Value	x	2 Score	=	0.2 Item Score
Total Weight: 100/100			**Overall Performance Score:** 3.35				

In this leader assessment example, this outpatient physician leader has an overall composite score of 3.35. Review of the LEM item scores reveals clear strengths in quality measures and lower performance in service measures. Physician leader evaluation and feedback provides real-time clarity of strengths and opportunities for improvement.

Weighting is a means to "prioritize" leader goals. Historically, physician leader performance goals are more heavily weighted on organizational quality measures. "Shifting" weights and increasing a leader's evaluation on service, growth, or financial measures can effectively help physician leaders "switch gears" and give increased weight to priority goals.

The process of developing accountability for performance as a system trait accomplishes several important goals. First, the visibility of performance down to the individual leader promotes measured outcomes. If a physician leader has a goal set that includes improving patient satisfaction and clinical quality measures, and that physician's performance is transparent to the entire leadership team, the effort to deploy tactics to improve measured outcomes changes entirely. Physicians care deeply how they "stack up" in a transparent, comparative performance assessment. Below is an example of an organization's individual leader evaluation reporting using the Leader Evaluation Manager. The individual leader pillar performance item scores can be seen by clicking "display score details."

Figure 2.5

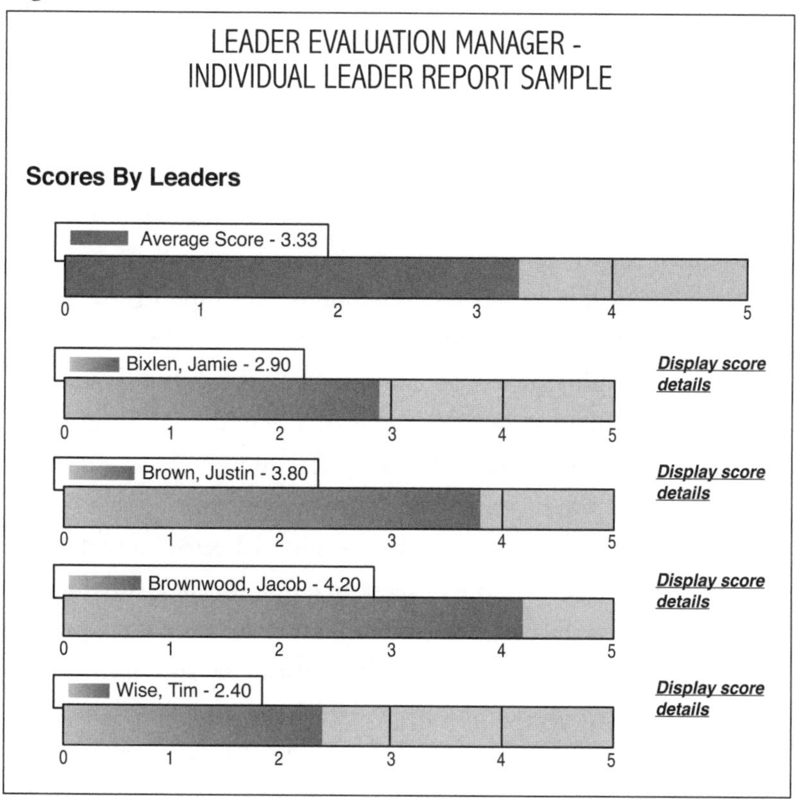

Second, the objective leader evaluation provides systemwide clarity of performance in real time. If there is a performance gap in the system, performance illumination allows for early intervention and correction. If patient satisfaction falls on a single measured group or unit, specificity of intervention can be done to address and reverse trends. Third, performance tracking and reporting allows for performance benchmarking and the ability to create incentive pay for meeting or exceeding individual goals. Pay for performance and leadership accountability move systems faster and will outperform a non-incentivized, performance-veiled culture every time.

A clear organizational vision with pillar goals, coupled with trained and accountable leaders, will lay the foundation for measurable results and meaningful change. Systemwide performance across pillars creates credibility for the mission and its leaders and earns the respect of watchful physicians. When a strategy is demonstrating outcomes, the outcomes need to be profiled and communicated to physicians. Nothing quiets physician critics, dilutes skepticism, and generates credibility and support more than pillar results. Performance matters to physicians, and the presentation of pillar-based outcomes will help enroll physicians to support and participate in system efforts.

I have repeatedly found that a leader's ability to get others to "follow" has everything to do with the opinions held of that leader. When a leader is not respected, has not delivered, and has no credibility, how can that leader expect to enroll others in anything? I was a coach, assistant defensive coordinator to be more exact, for my son's Pop Warner football team, the Wolf Pack. We lost our first two games. Our coaching staff received significant parental "input" and opinion regarding how things should be done. At one point, a public e-mail was sent by an upset father to every parent on our team, calling for the resignation and replacement of each of the coaches. The entire team was on the brink of unraveling.

Since no other parents stepped up to run practices for two hours every night, we kept our coaching positions. We stuck to our strategy, worked on execution, and kept the faith that our hard work would pay off. After our rough beginning, the tide turned. The

Wolf Pack gave up only one first down in our last four games and won our bowl championship. All the critics disappeared and parent support blossomed. As victories mounted, the same coaching message that had been vocally criticized earlier was embraced and supported because it was backed with outcomes and credibility. When a system is getting "wins," the leverage to enroll others is fundamentally easier.

Physicians want to be affiliated with high-performance systems, and the "status" of leaders in the eyes of physicians has everything to do with delivering measured outcomes. The paradigm of leader accountability will resonate with the medical staff. When a system CEO conveys to physicians, "Our leadership team will be assessed on its ability to execute system goals," it will transition physician perception of change efforts from the new "next initiative" to a fundamental and serious culture shift. Physicians want to work with leaders who do as they say they will, and hold themselves and others accountable for the vision and goals that guide the organization. Sharing goals and individual leader accountability with physicians elevates the leadership team to one that is intensely focused and outcomes-driven in the eyes of the medical staff. Physicians' respecting leaders for what they have achieved opens the door to a meaningful and durable partnership.

Key Learnings for Stage 2, "Leadership Development and Accountability for Performance":

1. Developing organizational leaders will position the organization to achieve results.
2. Many individuals in leadership positions have little training to effectively drive change.
3. An effective forum for training leaders simultaneously is a "Leadership Development Institute" (LDI) where leaders learn together on a quarterly basis.
4. The benefits of training leaders together include:
    a. Customize training to the organization's needs.
    b. Build team member relationships across the system through networking.
    c. Integrate physician and administrative leadership to develop common skills simultaneously.
5. Physician leaders should attend LDIs.
6. Develop a leader evaluation tool that reports leader performance across pillars generated within each leader's unit or region of responsibility.
7. Create "goal sets" for all leaders that are consistent with organizational goals.
8. Hold leaders accountable for results.
9. Report performance to leaders on their "goal set" on a monthly basis.
10. Leader performance should be transparent to the leadership team to increase impact.
11. Physician leaders should be placed on leader accountability measurement with specific goal sets across pillars.
12. Leader accountability and pillar performance should be communicated to the general medical staff to demonstrate a performance-based outcomes culture.
13. A culture of performance and leader accountability can earn respect and build credibility with physicians.

STAGE 3:
Establishing Physician Confidence and Trust

"You cannot shake hands with a clenched fist."

—Gandhi

The pathway to physician engagement and participation in organizational efforts begins, and can end, with the quality of the relationship between administration and the medical staff. Not infrequently, I have coached systems on physician engagement in which administrative leadership and physicians are both ready and willing to move on quality, safety, and service improvement, but each team stands idle with mutual suspicion of the other. Toxic relationships between administration and physicians will sink the best of strategies, and must be repaired prior to moving forward together.

When systems fail in physician engagement, frequently manifested as the opening of a competing outpatient surgery center across town, circumstances are rarely driven by money or market share. The diagnostic evaluation of a "divorce" between physicians and administration comes down to the fracture of trust, failure to listen, a broken promise, lack of leader visibility, lack of response to important concerns, and inadequate communication, frequently in both directions. Stage 3, "Establishing Physician Confidence and

Trust," is perhaps the most important stage in building physician loyalty and partnership. Establishing physician confidence and trust builds the collaborative, unified platform where physicians begin to step beside and into a system that has met their needs, kept its word, and earned their respect by the actionable items articulated in Stages 1 through 2 and delivered in Stage 3.

Any successful enterprise, in any industry, has been about the dynamic and the relationship between the leaders and the led, and whether leaders have created conditions that prompt, engage, align, and even inspire the workforce to deliver on the vision. The healthcare team, including members of the medical staff, is no different. What it takes to generate the loyalty of the team to an ambitious organizational agenda relate directly to the character and actions of those who lead the effort. The most successful companies, across all industries, have a cohesiveness of purpose, a unity of effort, and clarity of direction that are created and driven by their leadership.

How is it that Google was able to assemble the most talented programmers and engineers in the world? Was it because of stock options, pay, and innovation? Yes, these issues are important to talented, sought-after technologists. There was something else, though, that was distinct about Google that attracted the best. Google had established and widely proclaimed a mission to make a difference, to change the world, and to use technology for good. Its mission and vision spoke nothing of maximizing profits or market share. Talented engineers wanted to work for a company that was about doing the right thing, doing work that mattered, and making a greater positive impact on the world. These are the guiding virtues of the most successful company in the modern era.

In building high-performance healthcare systems, there is a sacred leader responsibility and opportunity to access the most important desires and ambitions of physicians, employees, administrators, and nurses—to make a difference, to do worthwhile work, and to have clear purpose in the care of others.

Effective physician engagement will be built on the foundation of a nurtured and cultivated relationship between physicians and administration. In fact, establishing trust is a precursor to any durable and meaningful partnership with physicians. The absence of trust between the administrative team and medical staff will make the prospect of moving forward together challenging, if not impossible. The importance of building trust with physicians *cannot* be overestimated.

The physician's role is central in improving health system performance. Physician support, visibility, and participation will heavily impact the outcomes and effectiveness of change efforts. Uninformed, uninvolved, and unengaged physicians are quite capable of creating resistance, digging in heels, and protesting worthy initiatives. When physicians display these behaviors, progress toward change becomes bogged down and utterly frustrating for leaders who are attempting to get strategies in place. The question is, how do leaders create physician receptiveness to change and a willingness to work together with the leadership team toward an ambitious organizational agenda?

In order to answer this question, leaders must understand and recognize the most important influence on a physician's decision regarding whether or not to step into a collaborative organizational effort. Physician engagement is a matter of trust and will bind or break the administrative/physician partnership. Healthcare leaders who proceed with performance improvement initiatives in the absence of a trusting relationship with physicians will have as much success as physicians treating patients who don't trust them. Trust in the leadership team *precedes* physician collaboration, participation, and alignment, and will be a vital element to the physician engagement process.

Press Ganey, a national patient and physician survey and research company, reported the experiences of over 27,000 physicians from 300 hospitals nationwide, between January and December 2007. From this physician survey data, a "priority index" was created to determine what was most important and lowest performing from a physician hospital practice experience. The results of this survey are provided to assess physicians' perspective, and to estimate what may need to be "fixed."

National Physician Priority Index Rankings

1. **Responsiveness:** Responsiveness of the hospital administration to ideas and needs of medical staff members
2. **Ease of Practice:** Degree to which this facility makes caring for patients easier
3. **Agility:** Degree to which hospital administration has positioned the hospital to deal with changes in the healthcare environment
4. **Trust:** Level of physician confidence in the hospital administration to carry out its duties and responsibilities
5. **Communication:** Quality of communication between physicians and the hospital administration

The physician's voice is clear regarding what is most troubling and most important to physicians. This rank order of physician concerns is born from the breakdown of communication, trust, and confidence between hospital administrative leadership and the medical staff. How do we fix these physician perceptions? How do we establish common ground so two groups can move together to achieve common goals? How do we mend a scarred history between physicians and administrative leadership that has the power to paralyze organizational change?

As in any enterprise, the willingness of the workforce to execute the vision of the organization is directly and intimately linked to the relationship between the workforce and its leadership. The relationship of the workforce to leadership is predicted by how the workforce is treated. Effective leadership communication, growth and development of the workforce, recognition for work done, and responsiveness to concerns build the foundation of successful companies and parallel the strategy for physician partnership.

As the executive team works with physician leaders to create and communicate the organizational vision and goals, the leadership team will have brought to the attention of the medical staff that something of substance is underway. The time to move is now. Long gaps in activity and communication can slow efforts and create doubt for physicians. Even if Stages 1 and 2 are perfectly executed, they are still just strategies awaiting implementation.

Building physician trust and confidence in the leadership team is the objective of Stage 3. Physician trust in leadership is a *necessity* for physician participation in organizational initiatives and support for a shared organizational vision. The steps toward establishing physician confidence and trust are laid sequentially to address the principal elements that will drive physician satisfaction and loyalty to an institution, build relationships with the leadership team, and clarify the physician's role in a high-performance care system.

PHYSICIAN ORIENTATION

The ability to convey vision, strategy, and culture requires dedicated communication and face time with physicians. A vision-rich, dedicated orientation can provide tremendous impact and clarify the vision and goals of the system and the physician role in the system's effort. It is much more efficient to proactively provide information to physicians up-front as they join a medical staff than to try to congregate new staff when they are rarely in the same place at the same time. The orientation is a means to provide system information, but it is also an opportunity to create a powerful impression of "who we are." There will be only one opportunity to do this, and the first blush with the system must *exceed* physician expectations. A physician orientation is a time to sincerely communicate an organizational culture dedicated to extraordinary patient care, superior clinical performance, evidence-based care, administrative responsiveness, and physician partnership as a unified team.

A physician orientation should cover everything physicians will need to practice comfortably, efficiently, and hassle-free in the system. The physician orientation session should be conducted by a dedicated, high-performing staff that performs all physician orientation sessions. Physician members of the medical staff should present components related to quality and service in order to increase impact and credibility, and to convey physician partnership, support, and involvement. It is important that the orientation delivery is consistent, the information is complete, and the presentation compelling. Logistical elements of this orientation can include:

1. **Introduce Key Leaders:** Introduce all key leader personnel in the system with personal introductions to new physicians. These introductions should include their training, expertise, responsibilities, and leadership results. Position leaders well to create credibility with the new medical staff. This is an opportunity to communicate leader accountability as a way of doing business and to recognize effective leaders based on their performance across pillar goals.

2. **Provide Contact Information for Leaders:** New physicians should have e-mails, locations, pictures, and phone numbers from key leaders across the system. Leader introductions and contact information need to convey to physicians, "We are here for you." Personal cell phone contact information for key support personnel would exceed physician expectations.

3. **Tour the Campus:** A personal tour of all relevant facilities conducted by senior leadership begins to build a personal relationship within a friendly partnership culture. Include the spouse or significant other in these activities. Physician perception of a system is impacted heavily by spousal perception and opinion. Leaders must sell the system and its leadership team to both.

4. **Provide Electronic Health Record Training:** Provide training and support for all electronic health record and physician order entry with longitudinal support for whatever is necessary to support physician efficiency.

The most important and differentiating feature of effective physician orientation is dedication to the organization's tactics, performance, vision, and culture. Components of this element of the orientation can include:

1. Vision and goals as conveyed in Stage 1. To generate physician involvement and engagement in system efforts, physicians must see vision and goals as the focal point of the entire organization and the depth of the leadership team's commitment.
2. Share individual leader accountability for goal execution. This makes a strong case for a performance organization and transitions from "we try to do this here" to "we get this done here."
3. Convey physician partnership as a core mission and trait for the system. Share physician satisfaction data and strategies currently underway to build and improve the physician clinical experience.
4. Share the administrative team's commitment to the physician practice experience as a system dedicated to its medical staff. "We are here to work together and support physicians in every way to provide extraordinary care to patients." Inform these

new physicians that leadership is fully dedicated to hearing the voices of physicians and to meeting their needs as members of this medical staff. Communicate the following strategies that they will see as medical staff members:

   a. Physician surveys: This is an opportunity to position the survey as an important measure and to communicate leader accountability for system response. (See pages 55-56.)

   b. Physician satisfaction team with physician membership: This team will be empowered to move swiftly, will report to the CEO, and will be accountable for physician satisfaction results. New physician awareness of this team will create credibility for physician-focused organizational intentions. (See page 57.)

5. Demonstrate the role of the physician in system improvement and share available opportunities for physicians to participate in current system projects. These projects can include evidence-based clinical protocol development, order-set deployment for common diagnosis, or patient service improvement. Plant the seed of physician engagement manifested by physician involvement and participation in worthwhile projects.
6. Articulate a system-based care model. System-based care using evidence-based medicine and order sets have superior clinical outcomes compared to the autonomous physician care decisions. Have members of the medical staff review order sets with new physicians, not as a mandate for "cookbook" medicine, but as a platform to deliver safety, quality, and superior outcomes. Position system-based care as an effort to improve the physician clinical experience, save time, and reduce variance in treatment for common conditions.

7. Communicate behavioral standards for leadership, staff, and physicians as a unified team dedicated to a shared vision. Do not be afraid to raise the bar, as standards of conduct are best conveyed up-front, and will seem justified and logical given what new physicians are learning about the system and its bold ambitions.
8. Provide a written summary for physicians as a reference guide that is given to all physicians as they orient to the system.

The intended impact of a physician orientation is to leave physicians excited about a high-performance system that is genuinely dedicated to patients, staff, and physicians. An effective orientation can provide mission-critical information in a dedicated session, and will begin the physician engagement, alignment, and partnership process. Equally important, the communication of tactics and strategies to physicians as to what the administration *will do* creates commitment and accountability for leaders to deliver on a promise. An effective orientation is an important beginning, and will open the door to physician partnership and enduring collaboration.

WELCOME CALLS TO NEW PHYSICIANS

Audrey Meyers, CEO of Valley Health System in Ridgewood, New Jersey, has earned physician satisfaction that ranks as one of the highest in the nation. In addition to conducting formal orientations for her new physicians, Audrey asks key leaders to contact each new physician with a personal phone call to reinforce a commitment to physicians and responsiveness to concerns. Executive leaders calling physicians as they join the medical staff will favorably influence a physician's perception of leaders and the prospect of working together. Calls take little time and minimal resource investment, are divided up among the executive team, and are logged to ensure completion and consistency.

Those leaders who establish a personal, sincere relationship with the members of the medical staff create the foundation for physician partnership and a collaborative culture that can move effectively together.

SURVEY THE MEDICAL STAFF

Surveying physicians is a tangible activity that serves the articulated goal of physician satisfaction communicated in the organizational goals. The initial step to building partnership should include running "diagnostics" on the physician experience. Evaluate what is going well and determine what needs to be fixed. The data collected from this process will lay the foundation for subsequent actions. The vision and goals created and communicated in Stage 1 include physician satisfaction, which is delivered in Stage 3. When surveying physicians, certain key leader actions are relevant to doing so effectively. These points include the following:

1. **Position the Survey as Important.** The highest level of leadership must communicate this survey as critical to the executive team's commitment to creating the "institution of choice" and responding to physician issues. Convey that this survey is the pathway to having the physician's voice heard, and to delivering what physicians need.

2. **Incentivize the Survey.** An organization that is in the early stages of the physician engagement journey should not expect physicians to jump when asked to return a survey. As leaders establish credibility with the medical staff as being part of a system that responds to survey data, physicians will become more willing to assist. Early on, leaders need to offer something in return for this important information. Something as simple as a drawing for a flat screen computer monitor is often enough.

Several commercial survey tools are available to assess physician satisfaction. An example of a simple survey is provided for reference. This survey was written by Jay Kaplan, M.D. Dr. Kaplan has over 15 years of experience as a medical director and served as Chief of Staff. He is a nationally recognized expert in physician operational and service matters. Dr. Kaplan works with me as a medical director and national speaker with Studer Group.

Sample Physician Satisfaction Survey:

Rate your satisfaction on a scale of "1-5" with 1 being "not at all" and 5 representing "all of the time."

1. I am satisfied with the efficiency of admitting my patients to the hospital.	1	2	3	4	5
2. I am satisfied with the nursing care for my patients.	1	2	3	4	5
3. Communication from inpatient units concerning my patients is timely and clear.	1	2	3	4	5
4. The hospital has the equipment I need to care well for my patients.	1	2	3	4	5
5. I am satisfied with the way test results are reported on my patients' charts.	1	2	3	4	5
6. Chart documentation and medical records (including space to sit and transcription) are efficient and organized.	1	2	3	4	5

7. Scheduling of procedures (OR, imaging, and lab) is easy, efficient, and on time.	1	2	3	4	5
8. The hospital is focused on meeting my needs as a member of the medical staff.	1	2	3	4	5
9. My overall experience of working in the hospital and caring for my patients is superb.	1	2	3	4	5

As a member of our medical staff, what three issues are going well or have improved?

1. ______________________________

2. ______________________________

3. ______________________________

What three issues would you like to see improved?

1. ______________________________

2. ______________________________

3. ______________________________

ASSEMBLE A PHYSICIAN SATISFACTION TEAM

Historically, we see health systems spend the time and resources to gather information regarding the physician practice experience, but fail to assemble a team that is accountable and empowered to respond to physician concerns. If a system and team are not in place to create a response to issues collected in the survey process, then I recommend physicians not be surveyed in the first place. An absence of specific, visible responses to physicians' concerns will only widen the chasm of physician distrust.

A properly assembled physician satisfaction team can be structured to deliver system response to physician issues. The physician satisfaction team should be composed of those with the authority to effect change and action, and should include physician members. The benefit of physician presence in addressing physician issues is two-fold. First, physicians will keep the team on track in terms of issues that matter most. Second, these physicians will position the organization well to physician colleagues as a responsive, "physician-centric" facility that is truly committed to its medical staff.

The objectives for the physician satisfaction team can include:

1. Assessing and prioritizing physician practice experience data (the physician satisfaction survey).
2. Creating specific responses to priority issues.
3. Communicating responses to the CEO, leadership team, and medical staff leadership.
4. Creating and communicating physician recognition strategies. (See Stage 9, "Recognizing Physicians.")

The directive for the physician satisfaction team should be to create a "you spoke, we responded" physician experience. Organizational responses need to be palpable and observable to physicians' concerns and problems. Leader response must be clear, concise, and visible where physician issues are followed by leader actions. Organizational communications to the medical staff should take redundant and duplicative multi-channel forms to assure physician awareness of the system response.

The outcome measures for the physician satisfaction team should include physician satisfaction, retention, and recruitment. Track and measure physician satisfaction over time, and make the leader of the physician satisfaction team accountable for outcomes and performance on his/her customized goal set. (See Stage 2, "Leadership Development and Accountability for Performance.") Directives and objectives for leaders without accountability for performance are ineffective. As in all action plans that set out to achieve an outcome, leader performance should be visible and tightly aligned to the overall system goals.

COMMUNICATE ORGANIZATIONAL RESPONSIVENESS

Remember, four out of the top five priority index "dissatisfiers" for physicians in the hospital environment were related to communication and responsiveness of the administrative team. Administration's ability to craft solutions and respond to physicians' survey results will establish the effectiveness of leaders in the eyes of physicians, and whether they have the attributes to which physicians will align and trust. The physician satisfaction team, reportable to the CEO, will be accountable for robust, visible solutions to physician issues. Don't be frightened; leaders do NOT have to meet every wish and desire articulated by the medical staff. What they need is to effectively execute *some* of the important items, and profile the solutions. If leaders solve the problem, but fail to convey and communicate the solution, they achieve little and establish no credibility. Profiling solutions is as important as the solution itself.

When physicians observe leaders who hear and respond to physician concerns, the seeds of legitimate partnership, collaboration, and trust are planted.

Several key points are important in creating and communicating organizational responsiveness:

1. Empower the physician satisfaction team to interface with different departments in order to swiftly respond to legitimate physician concerns.

2. Create a standardized communication tool to report system responses so that physicians will begin to recognize administrative communication as a trait of the organization that comes regularly and predictably.

3. Issue communications at regular intervals, even if there is no change in response. An honest, respectful conversation with clear details can preserve physician trust even if the answer is "no" to a stated request. Some of Studer Group's partners have issued a "Stoplight Report" (see Figure 3.1) to serve this function, posted throughout the facility and on the hospital-based intranet. The green column represents issues completed, the yellow column represents issues with specific actions underway with associated timelines, and the red column represents "no" with a clear explanation as to why.

Figure 3.1

REGULAR STRUCTURED COMMUNICATION SAMPLE: STOPLIGHT REPORT

Purpose of the STOPLIGHT Report: *To keep physicians informed of leadership actions to improve physicians' care experience in our hospital. The issues reviewed in the STOPLIGHT Report are based on information gathered during leaders rounding on physicians and the annual physician satisfaction survey.*

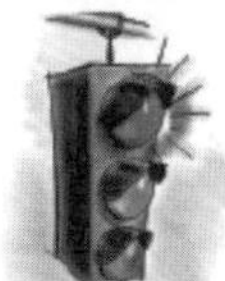

STOPLIGHT REPORT

Take a look at some of our results from rounding. More information is available on your department communication board.

GREEN/COMPLETE:	YELLOW/IN PROGRESS:	RED/CAN'T COMPLETE AT THIS TIME and HERE'S WHY:
Issue: Not enough parking available for physicians **Action:** Sixty new parking spaces added to the West side of the property.	**Issue:** Delays in the operating room **Action:** OR turnaround times study initiated with results going to surgical advisory committee for solutions. Will report actions in one month.	**Issue:** Expansion of ER on East side of campus **Action:** Extending property eastward is restricted by the city due to buried gas lines. Business development is looking at other options.
Issue: Comfortable and clean sleeping quarters for Labor and Delivery physicians **Action:** Bed mattresses replaced on all beds, and sleep rooms placed on daily cleaning schedule.	**Issue:** Delay in CT access during peak ER times **Action:** Additional CT scanner approved. Purchase and installation planned for next quarter.	**Issue:** Develop a dedicated orthopedic unit as a separate pavilion **Action:** Due to 42 percent decline in elective joint replacements in Q3 and Q4 of 2008, this project is delayed pending upturn in cases.
Issue: Adequate workstations for physicians on med-surg floor **Action:** Three additional computer workstations installed on med-surg.	**Issue:** Slow lab result availability **Action:** Two additional phlebotomists hired and currently in training to improve collection and reporting times.	
Issue: Healthy snacks requested **Action:** Salad bar added to physician lounge.		

4. Even though the system response is issued through a single communication message, the information should come in all formats. A newsletter mailed to physicians' homes, placed in the physician lounge, posted on the system intranet, and e-mailed to physicians blankets the medical staff and makes certain they know of the vigorous efforts underway to create the system of choice.

Surveying physicians and developing an effective, accountable, and responsive physician satisfaction team far exceeds what most systems do for the physician medical staff. These tactics are key in driving physician partnership, but lack the most important element to generating physician loyalty and partnership. The most important leader effort in building physician loyalty and partnership may rest in the personal relationship physicians have with system leaders.

The relationship with the medical staff cannot be developed from a distance. Leaders cannot lead and partner with physicians, or anyone, if they are not visible.

Although system responsiveness implies a sincere interest in creating a collaborative relationship between leaders and physicians, do not underestimate the importance of a personal relationship, one-on-one, between leaders and the medical staff. Nothing can replace this.

Dave Fox, CEO of Advocate Good Samaritan Hospital in Chicago, has earned physician satisfaction that ranks in the 93rd percentile and has grown market share by nearly 10 percent in one of the most competitive healthcare markets in America. Upon Dave's arrival at Good Samaritan in 2003, he described physician relations as "poor to mediocre." In his first two months on the job, Dave arranged over 50 one-on-one meetings with his highest admitters. Dave communicated a "win-win" sentiment for the hospital and physicians, expressed directly and personally by the CEO. How would a medical staff member feel regarding a CEO who cares and values his physicians enough to communicate, collaborate, recognize, seek input, and establish a personal, genuine relationship, one-on-one? Of note, Good Samaritan also has achieved levels of patient satisfaction above the 90th percentile for most patient categories, and core measures that rank among the best in the country. Physician engagement is a relationship business, and our most accomplished CEOs have figured this out.

ROUNDING ON PHYSICIANS

For two parties to walk together, side-by-side, toward a shared destination, mutual trust and open dialogue are required. Rounding on physicians builds personal connection to physicians and fosters trust with leadership perhaps more than any other tactic.

In 2008, I was presenting to the medical staff of a non-partner hospital during a dinner session. The topic was "The Physician Role in System High Performance." The physicians were engaged and found the information helpful in improving the patient experience, creating patient loyalty, and reducing malpractice risk. This non-partner hospital administration wanted this "unengaged" medical staff to "align." At the end of the presentation, a member of the medical staff stood up and said, "Thank you for presenting. The information was very helpful to me. Now can you train our administration to do the same?" He then embarked on a tirade of all that the "administration" had done to him over the years. This physician reported, with a crescendo of commentary, that in all of his years as a voluntary medical staff member, no one on the administrative team had ever asked him for his input, shared organizational plans, or thanked him for anything he had brought to the hospital. The anger and tension in the room grew to an uncomfortable level. Awkwardly, the entire administrative team was in the same room. The CEO made a relatively feeble attempt to justify the administration's efforts, but the entire room sensed the truth in this physician's testimony.

Ironically, this physician believed and supported the same platform of service excellence that the administration was trying to achieve. Unfortunately, he had so much disdain for the leadership team that the prospect and potential for a collaborative, shared mission to improve the care for patients was trumped entirely. Building relationships and establishing trust with physicians must be done as the foundation of all physician engagement efforts.

Can the hospital function sufficiently without direct leadership and physician communication? Clearly, it has been happening for years. Would a visit by the CEO to find out how things are going or a query to find out if there is anything physicians need, with follow-up tangible actions, make a significant impression on physicians' trust in leadership and its new-found vision and goals? Executive leader visibility and communication with physicians is a powerful collaborative gesture to build physician partnership.

How excited are hospital CEOs and members of the executive team about venturing onto the floors of the institution to take the physician pulse? This can be an awkward and daunting experience, particularly if there is a negative history between physicians and administration. Rounding on physicians is easier if leaders have a directive on what to do and how to do it. It is also substantially easier when there has been the communication of vision and goals, surveying of physicians, assembly of the physician satisfaction team, and visible responses to physician concerns. Physicians will sense clear change, and leader presence is a natural progression to the strategy and goals communicated in Stage 1.

Key elements to effective leader rounding on physicians include the following:

1. **Begin with a personal query.** Establish rapport, friendliness, and approachability with physician partners. Learn something about their interests, kids, and even personal circumstances. Trust is built on physicians knowing leaders and leaders knowing the circumstances, concerns, and aspirations of physicians. Be interested and sincere. These personal relationships and familiarities will make rounding on physicians substantially more productive, pleasant, and easier.

2. **Review purpose of rounding.** Some physicians will raise an eyebrow at leadership presence on the floor. Make what is being done clear to give physicians a "heads up." Position efforts in the following way:

"You may have noticed some changes here in terms of our effort to improve the quality of care provided to patients that we take care of together. One of our highest priorities is to be sure our physicians have everything they need. The best way for me to see how things are going is to come to the unit to find out what's working well and what we need to improve. Members of the executive team and I will be spending two hours each week to ask you and other medical staff members for your input and to share what we are working on."

---

3. **What is going well?** When leaders begin rounding on physicians, physicians may have seen the initial improvement efforts based on system responsiveness strategies. Specific queries will include the following:
   a. *"Tell me about something that is working well on this unit."* Use this introduction to communicate and share strategies implemented in response to physician concerns identified in the physicians' satisfaction survey.
   b. *"Are there any individuals I need to recognize?"* Physician identification of high performance by individuals in the unit can serve as an important opportunity for leaders to recognize staff identified by physicians.

4. **Identify areas or opportunities for improvement.** This component is the essence of rounding on physicians. This step represents a sincere leader effort to help. Queries would include:
   a. *"Are there any systems on the unit that could be working better?"*
   b. *"Are there any tools or equipment that you need to do your work more effectively?"*

5. **Round for a specific outcome.** Rounding is a fundamental strategy to get something done and to communicate organizational initiatives to physicians. Leaders may round on something as simple as reminding physicians to sit during clinical encounters with patients. Rounding is a key communication channel to convey what the organization is working on and to ensure that all individuals understand their roles.

6. **Use a rounding log.** When senior leadership rounds on physicians, accountability for follow-up and tractability of physician issues is related to documenting what is going well and what needs to be improved. When physicians see leaders rounding and documenting communications on a log, there is a sense that the interaction will not fade as the leader walks away. A list of physician issues will be generated and used as a template for follow-up leader rounding. Rounding logs can also be used to identify specific physician issues for the physician satisfaction team.

An example of a physician rounding log is provided below.

Figure 3.2

PHYSICIAN ROUNDING LOG SAMPLE

Appreciation — Input — Quality — Efficiency

Date: ____________________

Leader: ____________________

	Physician:	Focus on the Positives *"What's going well?"(Review improvement efforts underway)*	Harvest Wins *"Any staff, departments, or physicians to be recognized and why?"*	Identify Process Improvement *"What systems could work better and do you have ideas for improvement?"*	Repair and Monitor Systems *"Do you have the help and equipment needed to care for patients?"*
1					
2					
3					
4					
5					

7. **Recognize those identified in physician rounding.** When clinical personnel are recognized specifically by physicians, that recognition creates a powerful tool to replicate the recognized activity, improve staff retention, and improve the morale of the entire unit. Additionally, recognition of staff by physicians, communicated during leader rounding, will improve the working relationship between staff and physicians.

Recently, one of our staff physicians took 30 seconds out of his morning to pull one of our receptionists aside to thank her for helping one of his patients. The patient came in with severe lower back pain, and was having significant difficulty ambulating through the reception area. The receptionist saw the patient, stepped away from her desk, offered a wheel chair, and walked the patient to his car. This physician said to her, "Thank you for helping our patient. He was really struggling and you made a big difference. Great job, and keep up the great work." I overheard this receptionist speaking with her fellow receptionists about what this physician had said to her. She was beaming with pride, with a huge smile on her face. The impact of staff recognition by physicians is significant and can have notable influence on staff loyalty to the organization and its physicians. When physicians *earn* the loyalty of staff, the work environment changes, and the foundation for working together to pursue a shared vision is built.

8. **Repeat the process.** Leader rounding on physicians should be done at least weekly to assure interaction with sufficient physicians. The rounding log will provide the "agenda" and "to do" issues for subsequent rounding based on information collected from prior rounding sessions.

Leader rounding represents the leader visibility, responsiveness, and recognition that are at the core of physician loyalty to the system and its ambitions. The ability of the system to move together will be predicted by the quality of relationships that leaders, physicians, and staff have with each other. Effective rounding can achieve this end.

PHYSICIAN HOTLINE

Even "best-in-class" system responsiveness will have unanticipated operational issues and physician frustrations arise. The physician hotline is a method to capture physician issues in real time, before they escalate and undo much of the good work that has gone into creating the system of choice. The physician hotline is a 24-hour line available to physicians within the hospital when concerns arise. Administrative staff rotate being "on-call" for this hotline and are trained in issue documentation, communication with physicians, and follow-up pathways. Logs are kept documenting the physician, issue, and desired outcome. A priority system for follow-up is assigned based upon time frame resolution communicated to the physician.

The frequency of calls to hotlines is historically low since hospitals committed to this level of responsiveness to physicians typically have addressed most issues. When leaders have built a reliable and trusting culture with their medical staff, the need for late night physician calls is minimized.

The true value of the physician hotline is not simply having the hotline and the problem solving capability that arises from its presence. The greater benefits from the hotline are the genuine leader dedication to the physician experience and the elimination of issues that interfere with effective care.

Physician hotline numbers are placed in the physician lounge and within care units. They have dedicated posted contact numbers and communication to physicians:

"We are here to provide you with the best place to care for patients, 24 hours a day, 365 days a year. If there is anything that falls short of what you need, let us know and we will do what is necessary to make it right. Our leadership team will respond and communicate a response within 48 hours of your call. Guaranteed."

The hotline supports other physician engagement efforts reviewed in Stage 3, but should not be used as a stand-alone physician outreach. For the hotline to work, physicians should see and observe other physician engagement efforts, including leader rounding. If there is notable physician unrest without concurrent physician engagement work, a hotline may create difficulty for the leadership team.

The hotline can speak significantly to the main priority issues that predict physician satisfaction, including having their voices heard and having a responsive administrative team committed to supporting physicians.

PHYSICIAN PREFERENCE CARDS

In the spirit of creating a facility where physicians will preferentially do their work, it is important to actually know members of the medical staff and their preferences for patient care issues in the hospital. The physician preference card is simply a profile of physicians who bring patients to the unit, and what their specific preferences are in terms of rounding times, how they prefer to be contacted, and other clinical care issues. The preference card is a gesture that demonstrates a system's commitment to getting to know physicians and to ensuring that physicians have what they need to practice efficiently.

Preference card content would include:

1. Physician name and picture
2. Preferred contact numbers (in rank order) and preferred times to be called
3. Preferred rounding time
4. Contact e-mail
5. Clinic affiliations
6. Board certifications
7. Committee memberships
8. Hobbies and interests
9. Rounding preferences, including:
    a. Does physician prefer to round with a nurse?
    b. What clinical information does physician want at the time of rounding?

Figure 3.3

PHYSICIAN PREFERENCE CARD SAMPLE

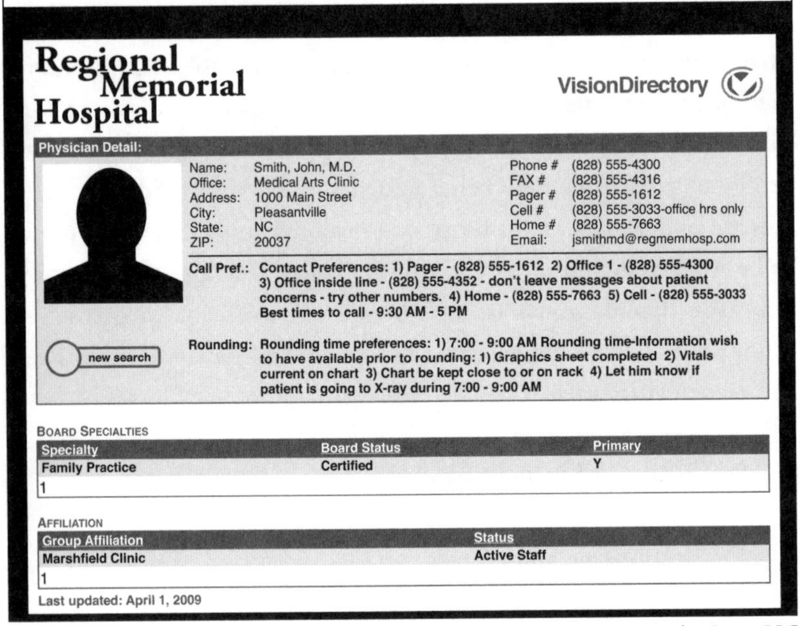

Regional Memorial Hospital

VisionDirectory

Physician Detail:

Name: Smith, John, M.D.
Office: Medical Arts Clinic
Address: 1000 Main Street
City: Pleasantville
State: NC
ZIP: 20037

Phone # (828) 555-4300
FAX # (828) 555-4316
Pager # (828) 555-1612
Cell # (828) 555-3033-office hrs only
Home # (828) 555-7663
Email: jsmithmd@regmemhosp.com

Call Pref.: **Contact Preferences: 1) Pager - (828) 555-1612 2) Office 1 - (828) 555-4300 3) Office inside line - (828) 555-4352 - don't leave messages about patient concerns - try other numbers. 4) Home - (828) 555-7663 5) Cell - (828) 555-3033 Best times to call - 9:30 AM - 5 PM**

new search

Rounding: **Rounding time preferences: 1) 7:00 - 9:00 AM Rounding time-Information wish to have available prior to rounding: 1) Graphics sheet completed 2) Vitals current on chart 3) Chart be kept close to or on rack 4) Let him know if patient is going to X-ray during 7:00 - 9:00 AM**

BOARD SPECIALTIES

Specialty	Board Status	Primary
Family Practice	Certified	Y

1

AFFILIATION

Group Affiliation	Status
Marshfield Clinic	Active Staff

1

Last updated: April 1, 2009

The forms of physician preference cards include laminated sheets at the nursing station, pocket cards given to nurses at the beginning of shifts for physicians with patients on the unit, or the hospital-based intranet.

Important elements to physician preference card rollout include:

1. Identify physicians for preference cards, typically high admitters or hospitalists.
2. For initial efforts, select physicians with positive nursing unit relations.
3. Conduct physician interviews to determine preferences. Simply conducting this interview will build physician trust and convey a system commitment to getting things right.

4. ALWAYS position effort as a means to providing efficient, quality care as a hospital/physician collaboration (get CREDIT for strategies deployed).
5. Create physician preference cards.
6. Train staff on application.
    a. If nurses make no reference to the physician preference cards while working with physicians, then the value and impact of the effort is lost. Nurses need to use information on the preference cards to influence physicians' perception of the unit.
    b. Nurses can use information on the preference cards to position physicians well in regard to patients and to have concrete awareness of a physician's experience and clinical background. When patients see that nurses know physicians well, it creates a sense of confidence and continuity in the eyes of patients toward the clinical care team.

Several important organizational objectives are achieved with physician preference cards, including:

1. Establishes specific identities of physicians who enter the hospital by face, name, specialty, and institution.
2. Reinforces a hospital's commitment to creating long-term relationships with physicians beyond just a referral source.
3. Conveys tangible organizational intent to make care easier and more efficient (a principal predictor of physician loyalty).
4. Allows nurses to get to know physicians personally. A physician who is treated like a stranger on the floor is a lost opportunity to make an impression and build a relationship.

"GOT CHART"—IMPROVING PHYSICIAN/NURSE COMMUNICATION

Though clinical quality of a hospital is measured by numerous objective clinical indices, physicians will assess the "quality" of a hospital by the effectiveness and clarity of communication between the nursing staff and physicians. "Got Chart" is a method to standardize nurse-physician information exchange so that quality, safety, and efficiency are assured. We know from experience that it takes very few ineffective nurse/physician exchanges for physicians to make the "generalization" leap to *all nurses* at an institution. The best healthcare systems evolve into a culture of high performance where tactics, strategies, and systems are built on consistency and reliance. "Usually" must now be replaced with "Always."

"Got Chart" is designed for nurses as a communication sequence when they call physicians for clinical issues in the unit. Nursing leaders will be responsible for creating consistent implementation for all nurse/physician interactions and for training staff for consistency.

Components of "Got Chart" include:

Before you call, ***did you***:

1. Ensure that you are calling the right physician (primary physician or consultant)?
2. Determine whether there are standing orders to cover this situation?
3. Review the physician preference card for when and where to call?
4. Check: Does anyone else need the physician?
5. See and assess the patient yourself?
6. Read the most recent physician progress notes and notes from nurses who worked the prior shift?

When you call:

1. Have at hand: Chart, recent assessment (all recent labs with times done), list of meds, code status, and most recent vital signs.
2. Enter the complete 7-digit phone number when paging.
3. Inform the unit clerk of your page to ensure efficient transfer.
4. Identify yourself, the unit, the patient, the room number, and the admitting diagnosis.
5. State the reason for your call.
6. Document in the chart: To whom you spoke, time of call, and summary of conversation.

Consistent, clear, quality interaction from nurses to physicians is frequently enough to make or break a physician's perception of a facility. "Got Chart" is a simple mechanism that ensures consistency so that quality communication doesn't happen most of the time, but happens every time. All physician relationship-building tactics deployed can be effectively unraveled by inconsistent quality of nurse/physician exchanges. Consistency with a nurse/physician communication strategy is a must-have and will validate the leadership commitment to physician efficiency and system quality in specific and important ways to physicians.

HOURLY NURSE ROUNDING

Building physician trust and confidence is not only about creating palpable organizational responsiveness, consistent nursing communication, and leader visibility. It is also about providing extraordinary care to patients that differentiates an organization from competitor systems. Patients who are more satisfied with their care in the hospital correspond to physicians having greater loyalty to the system.[3] Hourly nurse rounding is a tactic to improve quality, safety, and service to patients that will differentiate a hospital from those that don't deliver this service.

In 2006, Studer Group conducted a nationwide research study using twenty-seven hospital systems and over 2,000 patient admissions to assess the effectiveness of nurses rounding hourly and proactively on patients in the hospital. Nurses would check on patients hourly to assess position, pain control, if they needed to use the bathroom, and to be sure all of their possessions were in reach. Rounding logs were used to verify Hourly Rounding. This contrasts to the standard of care nursing model where nurses round on patients "reactively," or only when patients use the call light.

The findings of this landmark study are changing how nurses round across the country. Patient falls were reduced 50 percent, decubitus ulcers were reduced 14 percent, call lights were reduced 38 percent, and patient satisfaction was increased 12 raw points.[4]

There is nothing that makes for better rounds for physicians than to have patients rave about the caring, wonderful nurses taking care of them in the hospital. Physicians are more likely to support and partner in system efforts when they see great care manifesting at the front line.

DISCHARGE PHONE CALLS

Post-hospital discharge medical complications are estimated to occur in up to one in five hospital discharges.[5] Most of these complications are related to medication errors, failed follow-up, and a failure to understand discharge instructions. In a study of emergency room discharges, it is estimated that 78 percent of patients did not understand their discharge instructions, and 72 percent of those patients didn't realize that they didn't know their discharge instructions.[6] When patients are discharged from the hospital or ER environment, a system that deploys tactics in support of patient safety, quality, and service will improve physicians' perception of a system.

Calls placed by hospitals, clinics, and emergency rooms as a clinical follow-up to patient care issues have become a powerful strategy to improve the safety and effectiveness of the patient discharge process. Discharge Phone Calls are outbound calls made by a hospital or emergency department a day or two after discharge to check on a patient's condition. Discharge Phone Calls optimize patient safety, reduce 72-hour re-admit rates, reduce medication errors, improve compliance and pain control, ensure clinical follow-up, and substantially improve the patient's satisfaction with care.

Discharge Phone Calls are most frequently done by nurses and assess the patient by asking the following key questions:

"Hello, Mr. Johnson. This is Suzie, calling from Memorial Regional Hospital. You were discharged from our unit two days ago.

1. I am calling to see how you are doing. (This gesture alone will frequently exceed the patient's expectations.)
2. Did you make your follow-up appointment with your physician?
3. Did you get your discharge medications filled?
4. Is your pain better or worse than yesterday?
5. Do you understand your discharge instructions?
6. We like to recognize staff who have done a good job for patients. Is there anyone who provided you with excellent care while you were here? Why was she excellent? (Always harvest for staff recognition.)
7. We are always committed to improving the quality of care for patients. Is there anything that we could have done better for you during this hospital stay? (Patients love a system committed to improving.)
8. Thank you so much, and please let us know if there is anything else you need. This is my contact information." (Conveys that the hospital cares and that "We are here for you.")

The results from implementing Discharge Phone Calls can be transformational to the patient experience. Hackensack Medical Center in New Jersey improved patient satisfaction in the Emergency Department from the 50th percentile to the 80th percentile, and improved inpatient units from the 60th to the 98th percentile. Advocate Christ Hospital in Oak Lawn, Illinois, improved "likelihood to recommend" from the single digit percentiles to above the 50th percentile. Good Samaritan Hospital in Baltimore improved inpatient "likelihood of recommending" from the 5th to the 90th percentile with Discharge Phone Calls.

When tactics that improve care to patients are deployed, share them with physicians, using rounding on physicians and multi-channel communication to profile system results and create physician awareness. Tactics will have little impact on physician perception if physicians don't know or realize they are happening. Position Hourly Rounding and Discharge Phone Calls as tactics to deliver clinical performance, and share generated outcomes with staff and physicians. Nothing drives workforce enrollment and validates the vision more than measured results and effective execution.

Systems that deliver better patient care using tactics based on evidence will generate physician support and "proof" that a vision for quality and the patient experience is real, visible, and happening. System quality, improved physician/nurse communication, and organizational responsiveness are the conditions of the "conditional" physician engagement.

SUSTAINING COMMUNICATION WITH PHYSICIANS

To achieve and sustain physician trust and confidence in system efforts, communication follow-up is critical. A common leadership error is to launch efforts to build physician relationships as a well-executed, high-profile commitment to a new way, only to have it fade away with time. If this does happen, leadership's ability to credibly launch any efforts with physicians again will be significantly compromised. All physician engagement efforts must be built on sustainability. Physician orientations, satisfaction surveys, physician satisfaction teams, and rounding on physicians are not strategies to achieve a singular benchmark, market share, or physician satisfaction result. These strategies are a way of running the system. They will serve to differentiate an organization as something exceptional for physicians, patients, and staff. The tactics in Stage 3 are pathways for communication, and will need to be continually updated and renewed.

Several key strategies to maintain communication with physicians include the following:

a. Medical staff meetings in pillar agenda formats to keep physician communications consistent, visible, and aligned to organizational vision, strategy, and goals. Medical staff meetings are an important opportunity to convey current performance on quality, safety, and service goals, and initiatives underway to achieve goals.
b. CEO clustered e-mails: CEO updates and communications to the MEC, department chairs, credentialing committee, and other structural physician leaders that include performance and strategies across pillars can keep physicians involved in longitudinal efforts. Physicians getting regular updates from the CEO on activities, strategies, and outcomes creates an inclusive team effort and awareness of goals.
c. Physician rounding will serve as the sustainable method to reward and recognize staff and identify areas of physician need. Rounding is the continual one-on-one communication method with physicians regarding current system efforts to improve quality, safety, and efficiency.

CONCLUSIONS FOR BUILDING PHYSICIAN CONFIDENCE AND TRUST

Establishing physician confidence and trust is about executing efficiency, demonstrating responsiveness, delivering quality, and building relationships. Though building relationships between system leadership and physicians will drive physician satisfaction and loyalty, the most important impact of earning physician trust is creating physician willingness and receptiveness to *participate* in the organizational mission.

The process of building physician confidence and trust is fundamental to moving all physician engagement efforts forward. Physician engagement is conditional, and will happen ONLY when physicians' needs are met and when leadership demonstrates with communication and action they are truly committed to collaboration, partnership, and clinical performance. When physicians climb on board as a product of the deliberate execution of Stages 1, 2, and 3, the prospects and potential for organizational improvement fundamentally change. The goals and aspirations of physicians and systems are similar, and they need each other to achieve what they both want. Physician loyalty is earned and is a requisite for system high performance. Building physician confidence and trust is not only about creating loyalty to the system, but is also about creating a genuine and sincere interest in achieving a clear vision together. This vision can manifest when the administration's relationship with physicians is liberated from doubt, cynicism, apathy, and suspicion. The vision can manifest when there is clear and inspired benefit to physicians, the organization, and patients based on meaningful strategies delivered in Stage 3.

Key Learnings for Stage 3, "Establishing Physician Confidence and Trust":

1. Physician satisfaction should be a visible, communicated organizational goal.
2. Building relationships with physicians should precede all other collaborative efforts with physicians.
3. Use physician orientations to:
    a. Introduce key leaders.
    b. Communicate current performance across pillars.
    c. Provide all contact information, including e-mails and phone numbers.
    d. Provide a personal tour from an executive-level leader, and include the physician's significant other.
    e. Convey vision and goals.
    f. Share leader accountability model as a case for "how we run our system."
4. Assemble a physician satisfaction team that includes one to two physician members. The physician satisfaction team leader will be:
    a. Accountable for physician satisfaction results.
    b. Reportable to CEO.
    c. Responsible for responding to physician concerns and communicating responses to physicians.
5. Survey physicians and assemble a "priority index" for what needs to be done. Provide results to the physician satisfaction team as a template for actions.
6. Leaders round on physicians to include:
    a. Building the relationship (include a personal query).
    b. What is going well (review improvement efforts).
    c. Individuals to recognize.
    d. Processes that need improvement/tools and equipment needed.
    e. Round with rounding log for verification and accountability for follow-up.

7. Use physician preference cards to determine physicians' practice preferences and to know them personally on the units.
8. Use "Got Chart" to establish consistent, effective, "always" communication between nurses and physicians.
9. Deploy Hourly Rounding to create superior service and safety for patients, and communicate results and tactics to physicians.
10. Deploy Discharge Phone Calls to drive clinical safety, patient satisfaction, improved discharge instructions, and patient follow-up with their physicians. Share strategies and results with physicians.

STAGE 4:
BUILDING PHYSICIAN LEADERSHIP

"Great physician leaders conduct themselves as if a patient was at their elbow."

—Annals of Internal Medicine, 1998

When the vision and strategic goals are communicated and understood, systems are in place to assess and respond to physician practice needs, physician satisfaction teams are created, and physician rounding is frequent and visible, the conditions are set to move to the next stage of physician engagement and partnership.

With tactics thus far leaders will have created a facility that, from the physician perspective, is genuinely committed to being the best. Physicians will see that words are followed by actions, and that leaders do as they say they will. Accountability for performance as a system trait will transition perception from an effort-based leadership team to one that recognizes results and outcomes. Rounding on physicians will become easier as physician skepticism and doubt give way to collegiality and collaboration. The ratio of physicians' positive recognition of the system to cynical demands will shift favorably. Physician lounge discussions will change in color and will begin to position leadership as competent and responsive, and confidence in the system and its lofty ambitions will begin to grow.

Stage 4, "Building Physician Leadership," is about leveraging relationships with the medical staff that were established and cultivated in Stages 1 through 3 to assemble an engaged physician leadership to pursue a shared vision. "Building Physician Leadership" is about transitioning physicians from passive recipients of extraordinary service, quality, and responsiveness, to active partners where physicians have designated roles and responsibilities to drive outcomes.

Properly selected physician leaders will benefit system efforts, but perhaps not always in ways leaders may think. The most notable benefit of physician visibility and participation in system efforts is the validation created by physician support at the table. When physicians take active ownership, express support, and lead service and quality efforts, those efforts take on a sense of greater importance. System efforts become a top-down, cooperative, and comprehensive way of doing things, instead of a more distant administrative request. The ability of administrative leaders to implement organizational initiatives is improved and accelerated by the presence of physician support and involvement in change efforts.

I recently conducted a leadership development session on physician engagement at the University of Miami Medical Center in southern Florida. The medical center is relatively early in its journey and has delivered some very promising early results. At the beginning of the training session, individual leaders stood and spoke about results created within individual departments and how they were achieved. "Dissemination of best practices" is frequently the mark of a high-performing organization. Individual leaders spoke of improvements in OR start times and patient satisfaction. Each of the department successes included testimony of the involvement, partnership, and support of its physicians. None of the participating physicians who partnered in change efforts held any formal leadership positions, but each was a physician who stepped up to get things done, and the rest of the team followed the physician lead.

When physicians became involved, results materialized and change happened. Leadership was an activity and action—not a title.

The prospect of meaningful and sustainable change without the influence of physician leadership is daunting. The tactics in "Building Physician Leadership" are about effective physician leadership, physician leader selection, physician champions, and applying physician partnership and influence to execute outcomes.

THE PHYSICIAN AS LEADER

Effective leaders are passionate visionaries who are far more concerned with the success of the enterprise than the stroke of individual accolades or the pursuit of a personal agenda. Their enthusiasm is contagious and inspires workforce loyalty so colleagues become connected emotionally and socially to the organization and its mission. Great leaders are genuine, and the purity and intensity of their commitment to the system and patients enrolls and recruits others to follow their lead and become faithful to the organizational vision.

Those individuals who occupy leadership positions, yet who fail to impact the performance and behavior of those around them will preclude the organization from achieving its goals. The ability of an organization to execute physician engagement and cultural shift will ultimately depend on the selection, development, accountability, and performance of its leaders.

Jim Collins, author of the bestseller *Good to Great*, an intensely researched profile of transformed companies, has told us that it is not necessarily getting people "on the bus," as it is about having the right people on the bus. This is certainly true of physicians in leadership positions. The ability of physician leaders to generate physician partnership and performance improvement is about the leadership attributes of physicians who drive the effort.

Historically, physicians have gotten into leadership positions for diverse reasons. Some are approaching retirement and look to do something away from the intensity of daily medical practice. Others migrate to administrative duties due to simple "burn out" from patient care. Though good leaders can arise from these circumstances, they are not selection criteria that hold up consistently to attract the best.

In fact, one reported story reflected on a healthcare leadership conference filled with system CEOs and executive leadership. The presenter asked the question, "How many of you are totally satisfied with the attributes and performance of your medical staff leadership?" Three individuals out of over 200 attendees raised their hands. *Who* leads the effort is as important as the content of the pursuit. The attributes and performance of physician leaders make or break physician engagement and organizational performance efforts.

The "engine" of change efforts is the physician leadership team. Members of the physician leadership teams can include both formal and informal leaders. Both types of leaders play key roles in organizational change, and both must be "in play" to effectively leverage the influence of physicians to drive change.

Here is a summary of leadership positions, though they vary by institution.

Physician Leader Profiles:

1. **Structural Medical Staff Leadership:** This group includes the chief of staff, department chairs, division chiefs, credentialing committee, and members of the Medical Executive Committee (MEC). It is of paramount importance that this group of physician leaders support and align with administrative leadership in terms of organizational vision, goals, and strategy.

2. **Physician Champions:** This is a group of hand-selected and trained "champion" physicians who will assist in the execution of organizational quality, safety, and service initiatives.

3. **Informal Physician Leaders:** Informal physician leaders are those members of the medical staff who support organizational efforts, adopt change when necessary, speak up when quality dips, and expect other physicians and all team members to be in line with organizational standards. The number and visibility of these informal physician leaders increases as physician trust is established, collaboration is demonstrated, and confidence is built with the execution of Stages 1 through 3. These informal leaders frequently "appear" when a competent, high-performance environment is developed and physicians begin to believe in the direction of the organization.

Administrative leaders may not have immediate control over who is present on their structural medical staff leadership team. In fact, the executive team may assess their current physician leadership team and conclude that resistance within the current Medical Executive Committee toward change efforts will roadblock any meaningful, long-term collaboration with the administrative team. If these circumstances are in place, efforts will take longer and there will be greater reliance on champions and informal physician leaders to drive change. Alignment with the formal physician leadership team is essential, and performance efforts will be difficult without consensus and unity between physician leaders and administration on the goals, strategy, and vision of the system.

An important benefit of creating a vision-driven, outcomes-based organization that delivers a best-in-class physician experience is to create a significant *shift* in physician support for the quality, safety, and service system agenda. Both formal and informal physician leaders can be rejuvenated and realigned when Stages 1 through 3 are deployed. A new vision for the organization with effective, collaborative leadership can reengage even the "misaligned" physician leader by making the renewed organizational culture a significantly better place for physicians. When physician leaders see transformational efforts afoot, they historically "get on board" to provide input, participate, and "get credit" that comes from system improvement.

Physician leader selection, development, goals, and accountability for performance determine the effectiveness and performance of physician leaders, just as it is with the administrative leadership team.

PHYSICIAN LEADER SELECTION

Selecting and appointing effective physician leaders for a system will rank as one of the most important decisions made. The ability to implement strategy will be heavily influenced by the attributes and character of structural physician leaders. Are physician leaders staunchly defending the self-interests of a physician contingency, opposing change, and cultivating a "we/they" relationship with administration? Or, are physician leaders collaborative with system leaders, leading quality and service efforts where patient advocacy drives leader action to make a great hospital? *Who* leads the effort will determine how far, and what direction, a system will go.

Properties of Effective Physician Leaders:

1. *Effective physician leaders are driven by a value system that always places the interests of patients first.*

If this value system is not palpable within the medical staff leadership team, it will be very challenging to disseminate this foundational organizational trait systemwide. This value system is something that all great healthcare organizations must have and should be a non-negotiable physician leader trait.

2. *Effective physician leaders are progressive by nature and know what is required of health systems today to differentiate themselves in a competitive marketplace.*

Nothing is more stifling than to have a headstrong leader, who passionately argues for, "If it isn't broken, why are we fixing it?" Standing still in healthcare today will be met with eventual failure, and leaders must sense a burning platform for change, even if things are going well. Effective leaders must become experts in the rapidly changing and progressively challenging external healthcare environment.

3. *Effective physician leaders possess the ability to communicate a strategy.*

The structural physician leadership must not only have a strong commitment and passion for achieving goals, but must also be able to communicate and interact with the medical staff in a way that fosters interest, support, and participation for system efforts. Effective physician leadership is often about persuasion and an ability to articulate that a new way is a better way. Effective communication is not about mandating change, but projecting a future state that will be meaningful and desirable to physician colleagues.

4. *Effective physician leaders have the ability to create consensus.*

Creating medical staff consensus is easy to say, but challenging to do. The application of consensus in this context refers to several issues. The first is to create consensus so physicians collectively agree that the strategic objectives of the organization are important and worthy of pursuit. How physicians perceive goals is heavily influenced by how goals are positioned and communicated by medical leadership. Effective physician leaders should communicate with such persistence and credibility that colleagues will respond by saying, "I'm in."

Second, the creation of consensus is about a leader's ability to gracefully shift decision-making from a process driven by divergent individual physician agendas, to one that is steadfast and firmly dedicated to a system vision built on clinical excellence, superior outcomes, and placing the patient first. When leaders project a culture of "the patient is our only customer," the ability to achieve a shared agenda with physicians and administration moving together can materialize.

5. *Effective physician leaders possess the ability to stand when challenged.*

It is very important for physician leaders to listen and respond to medical staff concerns as they arise, but not to concede the values and standards of the organization. If a physician protests surgical time-outs, this should be a non-negotiable physician behavior that cannot be compromised. Effective leaders must be willing and able to stand comfortably amidst the heat of physician protest when physician behaviors run counter to a platform of care.

6. *Effective physician leaders promote the platform of system-based care.*

Perhaps the most important goal of physician leaders is to facilitate and execute the hospital's transition from individual physician autonomy to system-based care delivery. System protocols, order sets, and evidence-based medicine outperform individual physician decision making in nearly all clinical circumstances. The platform of system-based care should be a core principle communicated, supported, and executed by physician leadership.

7. Effective physician leaders are driven by passion.

All great leaders, from any industry, who create and sustain organizational culture change, are driven by passion. Passion is the fuel for deep, sustainable human effort. It would be a challenge to think of any great human accomplishment that has ever been achieved without passion for the pursuit. Passion is infectious enthusiasm and ranks as one of the most contagious of human emotions. To create consensus, push through resistance, and unify independent physicians to a higher purpose of caring for others will require passion from those who lead the effort.

Physician Leader Collaborative Behaviors:

Collaboration between physicians and administration will be influenced by the leader attributes of those appointed to structural physician leadership positions. Physician leader collaboration is achieved when the following activities and leader behaviors are observed:

1. Physician leaders meet with medical staff in support of pillar-based system objectives. To enlist medical staff support, the vision and goals must be effectively communicated and advocated by physician leadership. The most frequent venue for communication of system goals, strategies, and performance are medical staff meetings. If physician leaders populate meetings strictly with medical staff bylaw updates, attendance will be low and the opportunity to engage the medical staff in a renewed organizational direction and vision will be lost.

2. Physician leaders are willing to intervene on physicians' conduct that is in violation of standards of conduct within the institution. Silence by physician leadership when physicians participate in disruptive behaviors conveys that conviction for

the organizational culture is absent. The response to difficult physicians is a measure of the strength of leadership and depth of commitment of the physician leadership team.

3. Physician leaders position administrative leadership positively and communicate a shared agenda. Unity of message increases the influence of both physician and administrative leaders. "We/they" leader commentary is a property of low-performing organizations.

The selection of effective leaders is about leader attributes that are generative and can create followers who may not have followed otherwise. When leaders are identified, attributes should be used to screen individuals with leadership capacity. Selecting leaders is a long-term decision that will influence the direction and alignment of those they lead and should be made only when a match is found.

How does one really know what prospective leaders will do when they assume a leadership position, and will they be successful in leading physicians? Leader selection is about predicting who will have a high probability for success. When selecting physician leaders, the greatest predictor as to whether leaders can effectively lead is not necessarily their training or pedigree. Leadership abilities are best estimated by what leaders have done in the past. The greatest predictor of future performance is past performance. If a prospective leader has never undertaken or led a project, created consensus, dealt with opposition, created compromise, or pushed through resistance to execute change, that prospect may not be the best leader choice.

RECRUITING PHYSICIAN LEADERS

Effective physician leadership is critical to productively confront the breadth of responsibilities facing hospitals and clinics. Implementing evidence-based protocols at a system level, adopting electronic records and physician order entry, managing physician-hospital conflicts, addressing disruptive physician behaviors, standing as an advocate for physicians, and assuring the clinical quality for the system are just a few things requiring physician leadership. The spectrum of responsibilities can be daunting, particularly for medical staffs who rely principally on volunteers looking to make a difference. Recruiting talented leadership must be embedded as a strategy for securing effective leadership and knowing what works to attract physicians to this honorable post.

Strategies to Recruit Physicians to Leadership Positions:

1. Position the Medical Executive Committee as a dynamic, system-changing body of influence that will be at the center of organizational transformation.
2. Reward and recognize members of the medical staff for their participation and contributions. Place leaders on covers of newsletters and in the local publications to profile and recognize leader positions.
3. Waive medical staff fees for physicians in MEC or champion positions.
4. Invest in physician leaders and provide them development opportunities through internal leadership development or formal physician executive training.
5. Consider financial stipends to recognize physician time and leadership.
6. Provide benefits including cell phones, laptops, or support staff to more efficiently fulfill leader activities.
7. Issue press releases with photos for physicians new into leadership positions and publish them prominently in a systemwide newsletter.
8. Provide a parking spot with name and title.

Make physician leadership positions high-profile with impact and influence on the entire enterprise, who are recognized and appreciated for what they do. The visibility of accolades that come with a physician leader position eases some of the recruitment challenges that seem to occur with greater frequency. Make this position prestigious, dedicated to choosing and recruiting only "the best." Physicians who meet attribute profiles should be approached individually and positioned as one identified with the ability to get this important work done. It is tougher for a physician to turn something down when he or she has been "handpicked" for a position of influence.

APPOINTMENT OF PHYSICIAN CHAMPIONS

The physician champion, selected by physician and administrative leaders, is appointed to assist in the execution of pillar-based performance objectives. Physician champions work as an extension of structural physician and administrative leadership to interface directly in a training role with staff physicians. Physician champions are selected to achieve certain organizational goals, and will create the critical perception and reality that systemwide efforts are physician-driven and physician-led. Physician champions can be part of the structural physician leadership team, but more frequently represent the rank and file, front line physicians.

Typically, there is greater control over who assumes the physician champion position than the structural physician leadership positions. Who fills this role is as important as what they do. The physician champion will train and lead physician colleagues to create sustained physician awareness of the deep system commitment to clinical performance and the patient experience. In the end, the physician champions will help initiate, develop, and sustain physician behavioral change to execute service and clinical initiatives.

Which physicians are appointed to be initiative champions? Instinctively, most health system leaders think to themselves, *We have no one who is able or will want to do this.* It is important in the selection process to think of this not as a burdensome, thankless task but, rather, as an opportunity to have a prominent influence and impact on the performance of a healthcare system. It should be positioned as an opportunity to become an expert, a resource to others in helping physicians with important skills in which most have received little training. The physician champion should be well-positioned, high-profile, and whose role is clearly defined so physicians and everyone within the health system knows exactly who they are and what they do.

Selection Criteria for a Physician Champion:

1. Respected practicing physician who is well known and credible among the medical staff.
2. Is inherently interested in leadership. These physicians will have historically demonstrated early adoption and support for change efforts within a system.
3. Respected by nurses and ancillary staff as a physician who treats support staff well and is collaborative by nature.
4. High patient satisfaction. Physician champions need to display behaviors that they will develop in others.
5. Comfortable in speaking and communication, as many of the responsibilities of the physician champion will relate to speaking in front of others.

When creating a list of candidates for this position, the final decision should come from the consensus of physician and administrative leadership utilizing stated criteria. If leaders have access to objective performance measures, like patient satisfaction and peer review, these measures should be utilized as the initial screening process.

Physician Champion Responsibilities:

In determining who should occupy this position, it is important to create a specific list of responsibilities for this role. What the physician champion ends up doing will be a function of the structure of the system and the desired performance objectives of the organization.

The pathway for determining a physician champion assignment can include the following:

1. The physician champion can meet with physician and administrative leadership to determine desired outcomes for physicians across pillars. In order for the champion to be effective, clear benchmarks must be outlined. Most champion positions will have a *singular goal.* Examples of physician champion goals are listed for reference:

    a. Improve patient satisfaction
    b. Improve physician satisfaction
    c. Improve physician/nurse collaboration
    d. Improve physician-to-physician communication
    e. Improve specific clinical marker performance
    f. Improve implementation and compliance with evidence-based clinical protocols

2. The physician champion should report longitudinal progress on stated goals to physician leadership. The physician champion would meet with the physician leadership team to review current performance measures and action plans to achieve stated goals. Reviewing plans and results with leaders creates physician champion accountability for performance so medical staff training efforts never sit idle. Designated meetings between

physician leadership and a physician champion can be done monthly or more frequently, if necessary.

3. The physician champion will coach and train physicians to improve performance on stated performance measures. This will be the primary and most visible action and responsibility of the physician champions to accomplish system goals.

COMMUNICATION CONTENT FROM A PHYSICIAN CHAMPION TO THE MEDICAL STAFF

The physician champion will be an important communication vessel to the general medical staff regarding improvement strategies and organizational goals. Topics that can be communicated to medical staff from the physician champion can include the following:

1. **Communication of Organizational Goals to the Medical Staff:** Medical staff awareness of organizational goals and strategies is a chronic communication challenge for leadership teams. The physician champion can effectively review current system performance, future goals, and strategies underway to achieve goals across pillars. The following items are examples of topics for physician champions to provide to the medical staff:
   a. **System Clinical Quality:** Physician champions can report current performance and system quality goals. A respected physician colleague who stands in front of the medical staff and communicates, "This is where we are; this is our goal; this is the physician role to achieve the goal" is value-added and can begin to prompt and align physician behaviors. Examples include:
      i. Appropriate DVT prophylaxis using appropriate medications and/or pneumatic devices in medical/surgical ICU patients

1. *Why:* Patients with appropriate DVT prevention reduce risk of DVT and pulmonary embolism, compared to patients who do not receive prophylaxis
2. *Current performance:* 78 percent of patients receive appropriate DVT prophylaxis
3. *Goal:* 95 percent use of appropriate DVT prophylaxis
4. *Strategy:* Physician education, standardized order-sets, chart reviews with physician reminders

b. **Patient Satisfaction:** Physician champions can use patient satisfaction data to create and communicate a "burning platform" and a compelling case for doing things better, particularly if patient satisfaction performance struggles. Improving patient satisfaction and physician communication is the most common goal of a physician champion. The process of improving patient satisfaction begins with communication of goals, measuring and reporting individual physician performance, and articulating why patient satisfaction is vitally important to physicians (see Stage 5, "Training Physicians").

c. **Physician Satisfaction:** Physician champions may be tasked to lead an organizational commitment to improve physician satisfaction. Champions can report current strategies to the medical staff to create awareness of the organizational efforts underway to improve the physician clinical experience. Physician champions who lead physician satisfaction efforts as part of a physician satisfaction team can have a notable impact on the medical staff's opinion of the hospital and its leadership team. Communicating system strategies to improve the physician experience is as important as executing those strategies. A physician champion is well positioned to effectively convey organizational physician satisfaction efforts to the general medical staff.

d. **Employee Satisfaction:** Physicians care about turnover of nursing and the quality of nurses who care for their patients. Historically, physicians significantly underestimate the true impact of their own behavior on a nurse's work experience. Physician treatment of staff can be a core element of the training curriculum delivered by a physician champion. Champions can share the "plan" for training physicians that will promote patient safety, improve practice efficiency, reduce turnover, shorten lengths of stay, and reduce adjusted mortality. All of these important organizational metrics are heavily influenced by the nature and quality of physician and nurse mutual respect, communication, and collaboration.

e. **Malpractice Risk Reduction:** A physician champion may be assigned specifically to reduce physician malpractice risk. The reasons for malpractice events stem, most frequently, from communication breakdown between physicians, patients, and their families. Reducing malpractice risk as a physician champion training objective effectively aligns physicians and systems to a common and important goal.

f. **Low-performing Physician Coaching:** As system efforts progress and improvement in patient satisfaction materializes, physician leadership will often deploy the physician champion to coach individual physicians who struggle with patient or staff interactions. Coaching physicians is an important responsibility for a physician champion and a valuable resource for physicians to have available within a system. The criteria used to determine when coaching is initiated will depend on current physician performance relative to the goals of the organization. As physician champions are developed to coach struggling physicians, it will be important to have consistent and specific "intervention" criteria.

g. **Staff Training:** Physician champions who become experts in training colleagues in service and communication improvement can be an excellent resource for staff training. When respected physician champions stand up and train clerical staff, nursing, and ancillary personnel, the impact on staff behavior is significant. Physician-led training efforts within healthcare environments will change staff and nursing behaviors perhaps more so than any other training strategy. Physician champions training staff builds a sense of a shared mission and effort, and serves as an important unifying gesture of doing things together.

CORE COACHING PRINCIPLES OF THE PHYSICIAN CHAMPION

It is clear that most physicians have not been trained in elements of practice performance that are requirements for practice success. It is estimated that only 18 percent of practicing physicians feel as though they have had effective training in patient communication, though 83 percent believe that communication is as important as technical skill in creating clinical outcomes.[7] Building patient trust, creating patient loyalty, improving patient compliance, creating clinical effectiveness, and influencing what patients do are essential, trainable behaviors that are absent for many medical staff members. As a physician coach, I have found that physicians do what they do because they have never been shown how to do things differently. A dedicated physician champion will offer a systemwide resource to bring to bear core conduct that can become the trademark of the organization. How does one prepare for such a responsibility?

The position of physician champion begins with selecting the right physician using proper selection criteria and defining clear objectives for what they will do. Becoming an effective physician champion is about understanding how physicians learn and delivering curriculum that creates physician behavioral change. The spirit of a champion position is not the voice of authority imposing an agenda, but that of an expert resource to help physicians to be professionally and personally successful. When training is done with the right intentions, physician suspicion is disarmed, and receptiveness to change is built.

The following learning points are necessities for effective physician coaching delivered by an appointed champion:

1. The physician champion must become an expert in core evidence-based behaviors that will predictably drive the patient experience. Chapter 3 of *Practicing Excellence: A Physician's Manual to Exceptional Health Care* provides a construct of the physician/patient encounter and serves as a curriculum source. Stage 5, "Training Physicians," will also serve as a template for physician clinical behavior training.

2. The physician champion must spend time learning widely available information on physician behaviors driving patient loyalty, staff interaction, improving patient compliance, and malpractice reduction. The champion must know more on this subject than anyone, and be dedicated to constant learning.

Many of the skills of an effective champion are "self-taught" brought about from curiosity, reading, learning, and refining skills within their own clinical experience.

3. The effectiveness of the physician champion is about being a "like" colleague, in the same environment, who has gained expertise to help physicians. The identity as a front line practicing physician colleague builds credibility and physician receptiveness to the message.

4. When assessing and reviewing physician performance, physician champions should not render "personal opinion." Champions should rely on objective physician performance measures to determine a need for intervention and coaching. A key element of coached physicians "hearing" the physician coach is understanding the objective measurement basis of coaching intervention. Objective measures of physician performance in quality (clinical performance measures) and service (patient satisfaction) is a much sturdier platform to stand on to justify a need for change.

5. When training physicians, never provide behavioral training as a stand-alone intervention. Behavioral training as a siloed intervention rarely creates lasting change. Physicians undergoing training need to understand several training properties that create value and importance in the eyes of physicians. First, the coached physician behaviors provided by the physician champion actually work. Many systems, namely outpatient multi-specialty clinics, inpatient units, emergency rooms, and urgent care environments, have demonstrated that implementing evidence-based behaviors significantly changes patient perception of care as measured by patient satisfaction. A proven coaching method has greater influence on physician

behavior than a theoretical effort. Second, make the argument why this training is not about patient satisfaction or "smile school" but, rather, about predictable improvements in patient loyalty, compliance with medication regimens, reduction in malpractice risk, and improved clinical outcomes. Physicians care about being better physicians, providing more effective care, and having an improved reputation in the community, which aligns well with the outcomes of physician coaching.

6. An expert physician champion will learn that the precursor to physician behavior change is a physician's ability to gain the personal insight that *he/she* is responsible for measured outcomes. If a physician has low patient satisfaction, but blames others, or diverts responsibility, then fundamental physician behavioral change is unlikely. A core property of an effective physician champion is the ability to leverage physician performance data to *convince* physicians that it is their behavior, at least in part, that is responsible for their standing. When this chasm is crossed, then any physician becomes coachable. If physicians take no responsibility for their outcomes, then coaching will not change behaviors.

7. Physician champions must be fully trained in objective patient satisfaction vendor measures. A common position in which physician champions are placed is to "defend" attacks on the measurement tool launched by physicians who score poorly. Common physician arguments can include:

    a. "This sample is too small; this is not significant."
        i. RESPONSE: Set a systemwide standard for how many patient satisfaction surveys must be returned to use the data for a physician's performance assessment. According to Press Ganey, a national leader in patient

satisfaction measurement, an N of 30 is usually sufficient for individual physicians, over a specified time interval. The higher the organizational benchmark N, the more challenging it will be to collect sufficient surveys, but the greater the confidence that the survey results represent a larger sample, if a larger sample were to have been collected. Stand by the benchmark standard N. Champions should not approach physicians who have tiny sample sizes, because they can lose this argument.

b. "My patients are sicker than others."
    i. RESPONSE: The "I am unique" argument, ironically, is made by nearly all low-scoring physicians. Physicians will deflect responsibility with this logic fairly vigorously. The facts are that patient satisfaction and perception of care have never correlated strongly with demographics or illness severity. Two notable exceptions to this are important for physician champions to know. Younger patients tend to rate care slightly lower than older counterparts, and new patients will rate care lower than established patients. A champion will have the distinct advantage of knowing the literature in terms of what matters to patients, and what drives the experience, and can usually stand firmly on evidence to convince even the most cynical patient satisfaction measurement protests.
c. "Only unhappy patients return surveys."
    i. RESPONSE: This has not been born out by any survey tool measure.

8. Profile physician successes as they happen. As effective physician training is deployed, improvements in patient satisfaction will begin to materialize. The physician champion can profile physician performance improvement for others to see.

> Recognition of performance services several goals. First, recognized physician behaviors are more likely to be replicated. Second, profiling the outcomes of coaching and training validates efforts as worthy of time and resources. Physicians must see proof that something works to continue to commit to an activity. When a physician champion brings a résumé of improved outcomes, getting others to listen becomes easy.

Historically, hospital administration leadership has perceived chronic barriers and challenges to getting physicians to understand and participate in system change. The activities of the physician champion are intended to improve physician performance to achieve objectives, and to engage and align physician effort to achieve system goals. Much of the work of the physician champion is about coaching and training physicians as a physician-led initiative. Physicians leading physicians is an important and productive engagement strategy that is not possible with other administrative trainers. Physicians are more likely to embrace an organizational change when the effort is promoted, supported, and trained by a respected physician colleague.

CREATING THE PHYSICIAN CHAMPION POSITION

We have profiled the properties and responsibilities of a physician champion, but many uncertainties arise in crafting this position. How many are needed? Does this apply only to employed physicians? Does this position apply in an Independent Practice Association? Is this a paid position, and if so, how much? Here is a logistic summary in the initiation of this position.

1. How many physician champions do we need?
    a. ANSWER:
        i. Employed Physician Group: One champion can fairly easily cover three to four clinical sites, but ten sites are

too many, and will slow and dilute efforts. If more than one champion is appointed, it is best to select a blend of primary care and specialty physicians using the selection criteria.

ii. Independent Practice Association (IPA): There are pros and cons to this model. A principal advantage in the IPA structure is implementation of standards of conduct in a relatively small practice structure can be fairly quick if strong leadership is present. The disadvantage of the IPA is the absence of central governance to disseminate a systemwide consistency of behaviors. Physician champions who practice within the small independent practice must drive this effort throughout the organization. Physician champions must create consensus among physician colleagues. A single renegade, disconnected physician within a small practice will make change very difficult. In the IPA environment, success will be highly dependent on the commitment, example, and leadership demonstrated by physicians.

iii. Hospital System: Acute care is progressively provided by hospitalists in the United States, but many hospital systems still have an affiliated, volunteer medical staff model. Hospitalists or employed physicians (emergency medicine physicians, intensivists, radiologists, and anesthesiologists) are the first-tier champion choice based on availability and an existing relationship. Voluntary medical staff members who have demonstrated a commitment to the organizational mission, have an interest in leadership, and possess attributes to lead effectively can also serve as initiative champions. In the affiliated model, it is frequently a member of the physician leadership team (MEC) with strong system alignment and vested interest in the success of the medical staff who can serve as a physician champion.

2. Is this a paid position?
   a. ANSWER: Yes. A monthly stipend should be provided for this physician. The amount will vary based upon the scope of responsibilities and time required. Typical pay will range from $1,500 to $4,000/month.

3. Is there a contract?
   a. ANSWER: Yes. The contract can be an "at-will" agreement, in the event that unforeseen issues arise. The contract should include estimated time requirement (example, 4-8 hours per week), person or persons to whom the physician will report, and a list of specific goals articulated by the leadership team. A sample contract is provided to serve as a template.

Figure 4.1

CONTRACT FOR PHYSICIAN CHAMPION SAMPLE	
Position:	Physician Champion for the Patient Experience
Physician:	David Garcia, MD
Contract length:	6/1/09-6/1/10, renewed annually with terms of an "at-will" agreement
Goal of the physician champion position:	Improve patient satisfaction with treating physicians at Memorial Regional Hospital
Expectations for position:	Current patient satisfaction for physicians at the start of this contract is in the 31st percentile in a national comparative database. The goal of the physician champion is to improve patient satisfaction for the physician component of patient satisfaction survey to above the 50th percentile.
Strategies for improving patient satisfaction:	1. Conduct training to all system physicians in tactics and behaviors to improve patient satisfaction. This can be done in small groups or larger assemblies, at the discretion of the physician champion. 2. Report patient satisfaction measurement data to physicians. Assist in physician understanding of the measurement process, and be a resource for physicians who have questions and concerns regarding the measurement of patient satisfaction. 3. Coach physicians with low patient satisfaction one-on-one. Coaching can be done for physicians below the 10th percentile on consecutive quarters, or at the request of department chairs.
Reporting:	The physician champion will report a summary of performance and deployed tactics to the board of directors on a monthly basis.
Time requirement:	4-8 hours/week
Pay:	$3,500/month
Summary:	The conduct and behavior of physicians will significantly influence the overall performance of the organization. The goal of the physician champion is to improve patient satisfaction through physician coaching. The position of physician champion will have the complete support of all administrative and physician leaders. Leaders will communicate and clarify Dr. Garcia's role with physicians and his position as a direct extension of our leadership team and board of directors. Patient satisfaction for care delivered by physicians will be tracked over time to monitor progress.

The selection, development, and deployment of physician champions are essential components of generating change within a system as a physician-supported and physician-led effort. The influence of trained physician champions, with high visibility, strong leader support, and clear goals, can create shifts in physician attitudes and perceptions about system efforts.

Physician leadership and physician champions are the engine of change at the front line of physician engagement. Physician leadership is about empowering physicians to lead, harvesting their expertise for change and leveraging their influence to impact others. Those systems with effective, aligned, and dedicated physician leaders will execute their vision; those systems without such leaders will not.

Key Learnings for Stage 4, "Building Physician Leadership":

1. The effectiveness of physician leadership will significantly impact medical staff engagement efforts.
2. Physician leaders include:
    a. Structural Physician Leaders: These physicians include the medical executive team, department chairs, division chiefs, credentialing committee members.
    b. Physician Champions: Appointed to lead quality, safety, or service initiatives.
    c. Informal Physician Leaders: Medical staff members who support leadership efforts and the organizational mission.
3. Attributes of effective physician leadership include:
    a. "Patient first" in all they do.
    b. Progressive and able to lead in a changing external environment.
    c. Strong communication abilities.
    d. Consensus builder with the medical staff.
    e. Able to stand when challenged.
    f. Promote system-based care.
4. Recruit physician leaders by:
    a. Positioning physician leaders as principal change agents within the organizational leadership structure.
    b. Rewarding and recognizing physicians in leadership positions.
    c. Waiving medical staff fees.
    d. Developing and investing in physician leader position to improve leadership skill set.
    e. Considering financial stipends to recognize physician time and leadership.
    f. Providing benefits including cell phones, laptops, or support staff to more efficiently fulfill leader activities.
    g. Issuing press releases with photos of physicians in leadership positions.

   h. Providing a parking spot with name and title.

5. Physician champions are selected to lead specific initiatives using the following selection criteria:
   a. Respected by peers.
   b. Collaborative with nursing, physicians, and administration.
   c. "Profile" of the ideal physician within the system.
   d. Strong communication abilities.
6. Physician champion roles can include:
   a. Improving patient satisfaction.
   b. Improving physician/nurse communications.
   c. Improving physician/physician communications.
   d. Improving physician satisfaction.
   e. Leading clinical quality or safety projects.
7. Keys to positioning physician champions to be successful:
   a. Define a goal for the physician champion and how it will be measured.
   b. Create a contract with goals, time requirements, pay, and reporting.
   c. Develop and invest in physician champions so they have the skills and knowledge to drive outcomes.
   d. Provide clear communication to the medical staff regarding the identities, roles, and responsibilities of physician champions. The purpose of the communication is to assure the medical staff is aware of the purpose and responsibilities of the physician champions.
   e. Convey strong, unified backing and support for physician champions from administration, physician leaders, and the Board of Directors.

STAGE 5:
TRAINING PHYSICIANS

"Physicians go where they are welcomed, remain where they are respected, and grow where they are nurtured."
—Bill Leaver, CEO, Iowa Health System

After the system vision is communicated, organizational goals are set across pillars, system efficiency and physician relationships are cultivated, and physician leaders and champions are selected and activated, it is now time to work with physicians directly. Stage 5, "Training Physicians," is about an organizational investment in the most important player in the healthcare system.

The purpose of Stage 5, "Training Physicians," is to provide a road-tested coaching model to improve clinical care and the patient experience using simple, teachable, evidence-based behaviors. When a coaching behavioral curriculum is properly sequenced and expertly delivered, it can improve physician clinical effectiveness, patient loyalty, marketplace reputation, malpractice risk, and revenue stream. Physician training should never be positioned as a "patient satisfaction" initiative, but as practical and relevant training that will empower physicians to be personally and professionally successful.

If physicians are not trained and fail to embrace behaviors consistent with the identity of the system, then the system will face significant challenges in improving performance. Physicians are the perceived leaders of the clinical care team, and the care team will gravitate toward what it sees its leaders doing. How can we expect to create a system of performance and a culture of excellence if those of greatest influence are not demonstrating the effort?

Recently, one of our 12 clinical sites at Sharp Rees-Stealy Medical Group saw a precipitous and sustained fall in patient satisfaction. An experienced site manager was having a difficult time turning things around. I received a call from our CEO, Donna Mills, who requested dedicated service training for the site. We planned a one-hour session with the leadership team, selected nurses, and most of the site physicians. We spoke for over an hour regarding the importance of the physician leadership role, and emphasized that a turnaround would occur only if it were led by physicians working closely with the administrative team. Physicians left the meeting with a clear purpose, a renewed ownership, and a sense of responsibility for leading the way. Physicians and the site manager met with staff and other physicians not in attendance and communicated a recommitment to the patient experience. Physician leaders rounded on staff and physician colleagues to ensure the execution of service fundamentals. A sense of pride, team, and unified effort grew with a new commitment to be the highest performing site within Sharp Rees-Stealy. Within two months, physician participation and leadership helped transform care at this site as patient satisfaction increased from the 27th to the 97th percentile.

Leveraging the influence of the engaged physician who leads by example is perhaps the greatest catalyst of change in the behaviors of the healthcare workforce. Training physicians is an important strategy to not only improve physician performance, but to also create leaders and champions for a significant change effort. Clinical environments that change culture and transform results do so with physicians at the lead.

The ultimate measure of effective physician training is whether or not trained physicians change behaviors. Many "smile school" strategies fail to deliver by oversimplifying behavior change, and make the false assumption that physician training is just about showing physicians how to behave. The behaviors themselves are simple and relatively easy, but physician behavioral change is dependent upon a complex set of conditions and circumstances that "stand alone" training fails to address. Organizational vision, clarity of expectations, partnership and collaboration with leadership, behavioral standards, feedback on performance, recognition for doing well, and incentives to perform must be "coupled" with behavior training to make training effective. Drivers of physician change are sequenced, embedded, and developed throughout this staged manual.

PHYSICIAN CHAMPIONS DELIVER THE MESSAGE

The essence of effective physician training begins with physicians training physicians. The training message must be brought with credibility and delivered by those who have done it and who continue to do what they train. The extent to which internal trainers deliver training will be a function of the expertise and maturation of the appointed physician champions. Two options exist in constructing the behavioral curriculum and training physicians.

First, physician champions can train physicians using the sequenced training in Stage 5. This is effective if champions are comfortable with physician coaching and have been developed to effectively deliver the sequenced curriculum.

Second, bring in expert trainers to launch the initial sequenced phase of physician coaching. This is an option if there is a more urgent time-based need to get physicians aligned and engaged and if there are no internal leaders comfortable with delivering the materials.

If external coaches are brought in, several guiding principles are important:

1. Get recommendations from others who have seen the presenters before. You cannot afford a shot in the dark. Leaders need to be sure of what they are getting.
2. A physician presenter, or someone who has had direct clinical experience, is ideal for training physicians. Credibility in the eyes of the physician audience is important.
3. Meet with the presenter to be sure that the training is in line with what physicians need to hear and with what the organization wants to achieve.
4. Create three to four clear objectives that the presenter will deliver to physicians.

Once the training personnel is determined and assembled, other logistical elements need to be arranged. The most common format for this training is to assemble physicians together as a dedicated event. The duration can range from 90 minutes to a full day, depending on how much of the training needs to be done and the ability to assemble physicians. The training should be certified for Continuing Medical Education to increase the "draw." If physicians are employed, consider making this an incentivized event. Some organizations we have coached have shut down clinical operations for a half-day and have made physician attendance mandatory. In either case, attendance is critical if an impact is to be made. How this event is supported and positioned by leadership will speak volumes as to its importance.

Physician behavioral change is the final product of effective training, and will be touched by each of the sequenced steps of physician training. Communication training as a single event with physicians is not enough to entirely transform organizations, but it provides a sure start for changing what physicians do each day for patients, staff, and each other. The following steps for physician training provide a scaffold to guide physician champions and other leaders tasked with coaching physicians.

SEQUENCED PHYSICIAN TRAINING

Step 1: Creating Physician Buy-in

No behavior, and certainly not a physician's, changes without reason and logic. Physicians learn, understand, and embrace behaviors when they decide that there is a need to do so. The "threshold" for flipping the switch will differ by physician, with some moving very quickly and others taking a more protracted effort. Training physicians and providing physicians with behaviors that work is not the difficult task. The challenge is getting physicians to see the training as worthy and to use training as an effective and predictable change agent.

Making the case for change is about convincing physicians that a new way of doing things is a marketplace imperative and that failure to move can potentially have substantive consequence. The objectives of the first step of this sequence are to leave physicians with a sense that there is compelling evidence to support tactical behavioral training efforts and that there is a specific, compelling case that this effort is worth their time.

What does a champion say to make the case? Here is a list of well-established bullet points that are at the core of the argument for change.

- **What Patients Want:** A Harris Poll published in 2004 ranked the most important characteristics that *patients want from their physicians.* In rank order from greatest to least, important physician attributes included:

1. A physician who treats you with dignity and respect
2. A physician who listens carefully to your health concerns
3. A physician who is easy to talk to
4. A physician who takes your concerns seriously
5. A physician who is willing to spend enough time with you
6. A physician who truly cares about you and your health

A physician's technical ability to diagnose and treat a medical condition did not rank in the top six physician attributes that patients ranked as most important (it was number seven). The benchmark for clinical quality in the eyes of patients is based on a patient's perception of a physician's ability to communicate. There is *little correlation* between patients' global estimate of the quality of care and the actual technical markers for quality.[8] Communication ability is not only what patients rank as the most important feature they want in a physician, it is also how consumers assess a physician's clinical ability. In order for physicians to be successful, to grow business, to expand revenue, and to establish a reputation in the community, physicians must deliver the *patient's* definition of a great physician.

Are we not judged in the healthcare marketplace based upon our ability to deliver care and manage disease? No, apparently not. Eighty-four percent of patients choose their clinician on the basis of how well he or she communicates.[9] This is difficult for physicians to hear, and sometimes can provoke anger, opposition, and even disgust. Intense physician response is just what we want as we navigate physician change. Coaching is about creating focus and buzz, and ridding the medical staff of indifference and apathy. Physician buy-in for change is about creating an understanding and appreciation of marketplace conditions and the impact of physician communication as a *requirement* for marketplace success.

Even health plans are now leveraging patient opinion to help other patients make informed choices regarding which physician to choose. Blue Cross has launched a program in the Los Angeles basin in which new enrollees can go to the health plan website to select their physician. Patients can click on a physician to see training, experience, and a review of comments by patients who have been treated by that physician. The patient experience is a growing mechanism by which to differentiate one physician from another, and to help patients choose which physician they see.

Physicians' understanding of patient decision making makes the argument for engaging behaviors that work to influence patients' choices. The "case" for behavioral change will make the behavioral curriculum more effective.

- **Word of Mouth:** Over 65 percent of patients' healthcare choices are made by word of mouth referral.[10] It is what patients say about physicians to their friends and families that predicts a physician's reputation and traction in the marketplace. A principal feature of any successful medical practice is that patients become the marketing tool for the practice. If patients who see a physician do not recommend that physician to others, the prospect for practice growth and long-term financial viability is questionable at best.

- **The Physician Role in the Patient Experience:** The care provided by the physician in the outpatient environment is the most influential element in patient satisfaction, followed by the compassion, willingness to help, and promptness of the physician staff.[11] Physicians must realize their personal and significant impact on patient loyalty and their responsibility in driving the performance of a system in which they practice. Patients will stay or leave by virtue of their interaction and relationship with their physicians. Physicians who point fingers and deflect blame toward others for the patient experience *will* *not change* until they assume responsibility for their own behaviors. To be effectively trained, physicians must understand and appreciate that it is their conduct that influences the patient experience most.

- **Improved Patient Compliance:** Physician clinical effectiveness can be measured in part by the ability to create patient compliance with medical treatments. It has been found that the physician's attitude toward patients, the ability to elicit and respect patient concerns, and the demonstration of empathy each have an important impact on patient compliance. Conversely, short and impersonal physician interactions during which patients' expectations were not met have a detrimental impact on patient compliance.[12] Compliance rates for medications are consistently estimated to be in the 50 percent range, accounting for staggering increases in morbidity and mortality. The American Heart Association and a recent Senate subcommittee on medication compliance issues estimate that over 300,000 Americans die yearly due to medication noncompliance. Unclear physician communication not only compromises compliance, but can cause the entire medical encounter to fall apart.[13]

Physicians have strong feelings regarding their own clinical effectiveness. Physician training strategies should not be titled and communicated by leadership as an effort to simply improve patient satisfaction. This gesture will rarely fill a room, and can even turn physicians away. Effective training is done in the spirit of making physicians more clinically effective in order to drive better care and superior outcomes. It is far easier to enroll physicians in behavioral training when it is linked to clinical performance.

- **Reduced Malpractice Risk:** The logic for training efforts perhaps most firmly resides in malpractice event reduction. When physicians are made aware of drivers and predictors for malpractice risk, receptiveness to proven risk-reducing behaviors improves. Patients sue because they are angry, questions weren't answered, phone calls were not returned, physicians were rude, and patients felt as though physicians didn't care about them, listen to them, and left them in the dark. In fact, there is no correlation between the degree of physician negligence and the probability of malpractice events. Malpractice litigation is predicted by the degree to which communication has broken down.[14] Distinct physician behavior profiles seem to place the same physicians at repeated risk, with just 8 percent of physicians accounting for 85 percent of malpractice claim payouts.[15] It is the relationship between the patient and the physician, built over time and cultivated by trained behavior, that is most protective against malpractice litigation. Malpractice risk reduction is a powerful "sell" for physicians to adopt new behaviors and to engage in training.

- **Improved Employee Retention:** Thirty-four percent of all nurses who leave an inpatient position do so because of a negative relationship with physicians. Ninety-six percent of nurses reported observing disruptive physician behavior over the course of a study conducted within a Virginia medical center.[16] Physician conduct and interactions with nurses are important, and can make or break nursing workplace conditions. Respectful and collaborative physician/nurse communication improves patient safety and nurse satisfaction in their clinical positions. Nurses empirically have tremendous loyalty to and partnership with physicians, and the nature of the relationship weighs heavily on the nurse work experience. High nursing turnover prolongs length of stay, increases adjusted mortality, and can frustrate physicians who are dealing with unfamiliar faces. In the name of safety, length of stay, mortality, and the culture of team, physician training on nurse interaction and communication will occupy a place in the physician curriculum.

- **Improved Revenue:** Physicians with lower patient satisfaction are more likely to have patients leave their practices. We have found within our own systems that physicians with patient satisfaction in the top quartile have half the rate of patients leaving their practices compared to those in the bottom quartile. Losing patients is expensive. New patients can be up to ten times more expensive to attract than established patients are to keep. Established patients are more vocal in promoting a practice, more forgiving of service shortfalls, less likely to sue, and are at the core of a profitable practice. Establishing loyalty has little to do with clinical technical skill, and everything to do with the behavior of physicians. The prospect of "this is how to make more money" as a training dividend can make the curriculum relevant for even the most cynical of physicians.

- **Transparency of Performance:** Transparency of clinical and service measures can be painful, expensive, and embarrassing if systems and operations are not implemented to improve performance. Patient ratings of physicians on the Internet are growing at a blistering rate. Health plan publication of physician performance on clinical and service measures IS happening as we speak, and hospital quality and service performance are available at hospitalcompare.gov. In fact, the availability of this performance data is being advertised and promoted directly to patients in national media campaigns. The marketplace is being "trained" on how to use hospital, clinic, and physician performance data to make better healthcare choices. Transparency of performance will allow employers to pick the best healthcare systems and insurances in order to preferentially refer patients to higher performing systems. Performance quality and service ratings will allow Medicare to determine reimbursement schedules. Physicians can protest, complain, or ignore transparency, but it is far more productive to prepare for the new reality. Transparency is here to stay, and is a powerful motivator to improve.

- **Improved Physician Satisfaction:** I have spent a substantial amount of time coaching physicians who struggle with patient satisfaction. I have NEVER seen or met a physician who is indifferent to this issue. I have seen sadness, frustration, anger, denial, and dejection, but never indifference. Physicians care deeply about what patients say and think about them. It can be devastating for physicians to work at their craft for a lifetime and to sacrifice most of their youth to the rigors of their education, only to be informed that their patients are disappointed in what they do. Tearful physicians are a common occurrence in coaching sessions. Watching physicians change as they receive guidance and training for skills no one has ever given them is my most fulfilling work as a physician champion. Frustration and anger give way to enthusiasm and pride as the trained physicians begin to find the good in medicine again. Physicians are the smartest and best students in the world, and can turn quickly when they decide to do so and are given training on how to do it correctly. The correlation between the patient experience and physician satisfaction is tight—one will support and promote the other. Providing training to physicians in order to build relationships between patients and physicians is some of the most important work your physician champions will do.

Creating physician buy-in as Step 1 of physician development is about "making the case" and presenting the logic for change. When the buy-in argument is well made, the efficiency and "up-take" of the following curriculum is improved. Physicians will do what they believe is worth their time. The reality is that trained, consistently executed communication behaviors will drive every measure of performance that physicians consider to be important—patient loyalty, malpractice risk, patient compliance, clinical outcomes, patient safety, revenue growth and market share, physician reputation, employee retention, and the quality of a physician's work life. This "service" training is imperative to practice success and needs to be positioned in these terms. Physicians will ultimately do what serves their interests, and they must be enlightened to the realities of our consumer-driven industry. Physicians possess an alarming lack of knowledge and awareness of the current healthcare marketplace conditions. Illumination of these conditions in the initial training curriculum is important in order to gain footing for physician buy-in and change.

Step 2: Creating the "Burning Platform"

The burning platform is a real and tangible internal performance issue that makes the argument and drives urgency for change. One could argue that organizational change in the absence of a burning platform is far slower, and frequently doesn't happen at all. Step 2 is about lifting the hood and illuminating organizational reality that creates a very specific and meaningful "call to action."

This step can be a source of physician emotion, conviction, and intense response. In the absence of these human emotions, the initiation of change takes far more effort. Emotions are the strongest driver behind behavioral change, and effective champions will leverage this reality in coaching physicians.

A compelling burning platform can ignite a transformational systemwide change. The Urgent Care Centers at the Sharp Rees-Stealy Medical Group in San Diego is a busy system, having over

150,000 patient visits per year. In our remote past, our urgent care struggled with the patient experience. In fact, it was not uncommon for urgent care to be in the single percentiles in a national database for patient satisfaction. As the rest of our system was moving forward with performance improvement, it was clear that urgent care had to change.

In an attempt to determine the source of patient sentiment, our leadership team ran a "diagnostic" evaluation of patients' experiences in urgent care. Our leadership team was aware of the importance of pain management as an important contributor to the overall patient experience, and that is where our team looked.

Pain management was evaluated by how frequently patients who came into urgent care with a pain complaint were assessed and treated for their pain during their visit. Chest and abdominal pain patients were excluded. Prior to acquiring data on pain management performance, urgent care physicians were informally queried on their ability to effectively manage pain. Leaders asked physicians, "How are you doing in managing pain?" In the absence of actual data measurement, physicians' empiric self-assessment was that they were "pretty good" when it came to assessing and treating pain.

One hundred twenty charts were pulled and manually reviewed (this was prior to the electronic health record). Of all the charts that were pulled, 11 patients out of 120 were assessed and treated for their pain. The reality of urgent care performance was in stark contrast to physicians' opinion of themselves. In the absence of reflective performance data and when self-perception of care is "pretty good," there is little logic or drive to do things differently.

In report after report and case after case, pain conditions were left unassessed, untreated, and uncared for in urgent care. Fractures, back injuries, and broken noses came and went with no queries as to the patient's pain, and no effort to make it better. During an urgent care leadership meeting that followed, the pain management data was presented. The room fell silent. Bill Christiansen, a prominent physician leader who stands well over 6 feet, heard the data, stood from his chair, and looked at everyone in the room. "This will not be happening here anymore." The burning platform was on fire. Door to doc times were established, Discharge Phone Calls were deployed, keeping patients informed of waits was hardwired, and a pain management protocol was launched to assess and treat patients at the door for their pain. The Sharp Rees-Stealy Medical Group Urgent Care System has now been recognized at a national level for its transformational turnaround in service and quality, and ranks at the top of the database for pain management and the patient experience.

Burning platforms can take several forms, but the common link between burning platforms that generate impact are those that stir response, discussion, and emotion. A 1 percent loss of market share will not have impact on physicians or change behavior. Transparently reported patient experience data dialed down to individual units or to individual physicians has impact. A sentinel event in which a patient under system care is harmed through communication breakdown or human error has impact.

Every system, no matter how good, has meaningful events or performance data that speaks to physicians. Creating buy-in with a logical, compelling case for the benefit of change, coupled to a credible case or to data that demands change, can position training as worthy and necessary. Again, it is not the training that occurs in a silo, but the training in the context of other drivers of change that makes training effective.

Step 3: Behavioral Training for Physicians

Creating buy-in and urgency will provide logic and relevance for the "how-to" behavioral curriculum that will follow in Step 3. The behavioral training itself is prescriptive and easy to do, but physicians will begin to embed these behaviors only if there is a clear need and benefit for them and for patients.

At Studer Group, we use a systemic training method of communication that is used for physicians, nurses, ancillary personnel, and administrative leadership. The training used to transform the healthcare experience is referred to as AIDET®. AIDET is an acronym that represents the framework to effective communication with patients and will be presented in the context of physician training:

A is for *acknowledge:* how physicians greet patients and establish a first impression

I is for *introduce:* how physicians and others introduce themselves to patients, their roles on the care team, and the experience and expertise brought to a case

D is for *duration:* keeping patients informed on wait times, admission length, test turnaround times, therapeutic effect, or symptom resolution

E is for *explanation:* providing patients with information on treatment, medications, diagnosis, and therapy options

T is for *thank you:* thanking patients for trusting physicians with their care as well as closing the clinical encounter

As a consistent "always" form of communication, AIDET is road tested and has been proven to work in virtually every healthcare environment. There is now extensive experience in the application of AIDET in emergency departments, inpatient units, outpatient clinics, urgent cares, nursing homes, occupational health clinics, and hospice systems. AIDET can be presented and specified for physicians in order to deliver on a system commitment to service, safety, and outcomes. AIDET will be the scaffold for systemwide training, so that there is consistency of training methods for those treating patients.

Training physicians in AIDET is part of the continuum of system development consistent with the stated vision and goals of the organization. The intended outcome of AIDET behaviors will certainly improve the patient perception of care and create measurable change in patient satisfaction, but there are other, more clinically important outcomes from an *always* AIDET culture. Patients will take medications, comply with treatment regimens, have less anxiety, follow recommendations, and better execute discharge instructions. Training and implementing AIDET "operationalizes" compassion and communication, builds patient loyalty, drives outcomes, and provides physicians and the entire team proven tools to improve patient care.

AIDET will be segmented into its individual components so that it applies to physicians in a meaningful, practical, and simple way. AIDET is the behavioral curriculum for training physicians and can be delivered by selected physician champions, physician leaders, and experts in coaching AIDET.

ACKNOWLEDGE

How physicians greet and acknowledge patients can position the encounter effectively or can tarnish a first impression from which it can be difficult to recover. Patients are frequently anxiously awaiting the physician in healthcare environments and are keenly perceptive as to the verbal and nonverbal communications during the initial seconds of the encounter. It will be critical for physicians to do this well.

Important elements for *acknowledging* patients include:

- Physicians should be aware of relevant clinical data *prior* to seeing the patient. Nothing fractures the patient trust more than a physician who walks into a clinical encounter blinded by ignorance of important patient information. Physicians need to know and communicate to the patient an awareness of relevant clinical events, consult opinions, diagnostic test results, and what they have done during prior encounters with the patient.

- Knock on the door prior to entry. This is out of simple respect for patient apprehension and conveys respect for the patient's privacy. The knock should be followed by a brief two-second pause prior to entry.
- Look at the patient and make eye contact upon entering the room. Frequently, family members or a friend will be with the patient, and it is important to establish clear contact and acknowledgment of them as well. A physician who ignores family or friends in the room will establish a negative initial impression that will be difficult to resurrect.
- Use the patient's name. Recent studies have demonstrated that physicians will use the patient's name less than 50 percent of the time during clinical encounters.[17] Medical errors occur by failing to identify patients properly, and using the patient's name is a means to assure proper patient identification in addition to providing a personalized touch.
- Smile and shake the patient's hand. The impact of the human touch should not be underestimated. A physician who gestures with a smile, faces the patient, and greets the patient by name creates physician "approachability." Depressed, withdrawn, reclusive, and frustrated physicians are easy for patients to spot and can create a "disconnect" in the opening seconds of the encounter.
- Sit at the patient's level for the clinical encounter. Physicians who sit are assessed by patients as spending more time and having greater compassion than those physicians who do not sit.[18] Important nonverbal communication actions for physicians to exhibit include leaning forward, facing the patient, and using hand expressions with palms up. These movements convey physician concern and kindness as well as a physician

commitment to caring for and listening to the patient. Body language has a significant influence on the patient's perception of a physician in the first moments of the encounter, and physician awareness of this is an important component of behavioral training.

- First impressions are also generated by the appearance of a facility. Reception areas should be spotless with current reading materials. Receptionists should be friendly and genuine, and treat each patient as they enter the facility as though they were waiting for them, specifically.
- Acknowledge patients and fellow team members in the halls of your facility. Eye contact, a smile, and a "hello" from *everyone* wearing an ID badge as patients and families walk your facility creates a favorable impression and speaks to the "character" of the institution.

The first seconds in *acknowledge* must convey clinical confidence, approachability, compassion, and kindness from a physician who genuinely cares about patients. Most physicians agree that properly acknowledging patients is important and can significantly impact patient perception. Unfortunately, these same physicians are frequently running behind, rushed with large clinical loads, and can easily fall into prior ways of doing things. The key elements to effective physician training are the importance of consistency and executing behaviors in all circumstances. The difference between the good and the great in the eyes of the patient marketplace lies in those physicians who can be relied on to always do certain things, and the patient comfort and confidence that come from a reliable and predictable experience.

AIDET applies to every member of the team, and physicians will expect to see training as a systemwide effort. Though physicians should be involved early in organizational change efforts, they should never be trained in the absence of their support staff. Nothing will frustrate physicians more than making a personal commitment to improving care and communication to patients, only to see nurses and receptionists failing to do the same.

INTRODUCE

In January 2009, a study published in *The Archives of Internal Medicine* reported that 75 percent of patients admitted to a university of Chicago hospital were unable to name a single doctor assigned to their care. Of the remaining 25 percent who were able to give a name, only 40 percent were correct.

A well-executed physician introduction can place a patient at ease, reduce patient anxiety, and solidify a patient's first impression.

Key elements to *introduction* for physicians include the following:

- The physician should introduce himself/herself by name. Several options exist here. Contrary to historical instructions, studies have found that the patient-preferred method of introduction is the physician's first and last name.[19] The first and last name reduces formality and improves physician approachability. Consider this component to be a personal choice and style for physicians in terms of the title they use to introduce themselves.

- Physicians should describe their exact role in the care of the patient. Physicians should *never assume* that the patient knows this key piece of information. The average patient can encounter nearly 30 care providers following surgical admission and 20 providers for medical cases.[20] The absence of clear introductions can instill confusion, provoke anxiety, and diminish trust as patients wonder who these physicians are and what they are supposed to be doing.

At the time this manual was being written, my mother-in-law was discharged to her home after a protracted hospital stay for a ruptured esophagus repair. The care she received at our main Sharp Memorial Campus was excellent. My wife was there with her mom every day. AIDET was delivered at nearly every interaction as nurses, hospitalists, and surgeons cared expertly for the patient. On one occasion during her three-week hospitalization, a respiratory therapist failed to introduce herself and her role in the care team. She abruptly hooked up an albuterol nebulized treatment and stood in silence as my mother-in-law breathed in and out of the mask pressed to her face. My wife is not in the medical field, and had no idea of who the respiratory therapist was or what she was doing. My wife called me, anxious and concerned about the bedside activity. I explained what was happening, but her confidence and trust in the team took a step back because a single care provider did not introduce herself to the patient and the family. It took several days before my wife felt at ease leaving her mother alone. Clear and consistent introductions to patients and families are important.

- Physicians should communicate their experience and expertise. Patients want to know that a physician has experience and they are in competent, expert hands. If a surgeon consents a patient for a routine laparoscopic cholecystectomy, the patient *hopes* that the surgeon is experienced and well trained. If that same surgeon says he has been doing this procedure for over 15 years and has completed thousands of laparoscopic cholecystectomies, the patient *knows* that he or she is in expert hands. Confidence is built, anxiety is reduced, and patient perception is improved. Physicians positioning themselves, fellow physicians, staff members, departments, or the system well is referred to as "managing up." Managing up is a powerful technique that improves patient perception of physicians, staff, and departments, and is an easily trained physician behavior.

An effective introduction can look like this:

"Mrs. Smith, nice to meet you. My name is Stewart Jacobs, and I am the hospitalist physician who will be taking care of you tonight. I work with your primary care physician, Dr. Spees, and specialize in taking care of patients who require care in the hospital. I am the chairman of the hospitalist program and have been taking care of patients here for over seven years. Our hospitalist physicians are in the hospital 24 hours a day to make sure that you have everything you need to get better, faster."

A properly executed physician introduction can take advantage of the unique physician influence on patient perception. Patients are attentive, and will remember clearly what physicians say about others on the clinical care team. If our hospitalist, Stewart Jacobs, were trained on how to apply managing up he could effectively pave the way for the rest of the care team through several tactical communications:

- *"Dr. Spees is an outstanding family medicine physician. I have known him for years, and you are lucky to be in his care."*
- *"Susie will be your nurse tonight. You are in excellent hands. She is one of our best."*

Managing up takes very little time and is proven to reduce patient anxiety and improve perception of care. When physicians begin to position nurses and colleagues well, patients begin to talk. A patient will say to a nurse that Dr. Jacobs mentioned that she was one of the best. What does that patient comment do to the dynamic between the nurse and physician? Systemic efforts to train and implement managing up can begin to shift cultures of healthcare systems to a collaborative, collegial, and cooperative team that works together to take great care of patients.

DURATION

Providing information to patients regarding "duration" is at the core of the healthcare experience. Every contact point for patients involves a wait for something. How long until the test results return? How long until the biopsy is interpreted? How long until the MRI is completed? How long until the patient is seen by the physician? Systems and physicians who are best-in-class keep patients informed all of the time.

Wait Time Durations: Overall patient satisfaction drops in a linear fashion according to wait times. Press Ganey, a patient satisfaction survey company that runs the largest comparative database in the country, looks specifically at wait times and how they correspond to overall patient satisfaction in the outpatient and emergency room environments. In 2006, Press Ganey reviewed nearly two million outpatient encounters from 1,100 facilities. Those encounters with wait times of 15 minutes or less scored substantially higher than those with longer wait times. More specifically, those with wait times under 15 minutes scored above the 80th percentile, while those encounters with wait times over an hour scored in the 1st percentile.[21]

The correlation between wait times and patient satisfaction is significant. Within this data set, the impact of keeping patients informed of wait times on patients' overall perception of care is most compelling. Reviewing Press Ganey's patient satisfaction data from 1,552 emergency departments in 2006, patient satisfaction was at the top of the database even when wait times exceeded four hours if patients rated "how well were you kept informed about delays" as "very good" (the highest rating). Conversely, even with wait times of less than one hour, patients rated emergency departments low in patient satisfaction if the patient assessment of "how well were you kept informed about delays" was also rated low. The patient perception was driven more by how well patients were kept informed than by the wait time itself. Keeping patients informed of wait times and durations is an essential tactic in preserving the patient experience, particularly in challenging workflow environments when wait times may be long.

Diagnostic Testing Durations: Patients who are kept well informed call less frequently, complain less, and are more satisfied with every element of care. Providing information regarding the duration of time and waits manages patient expectations and reduces workload for physicians and healthcare systems. Additional training components for physician communication regarding duration include the following:

1. *Physicians should inform patients of how long the hospital stay is likely to be.* This is what patients want to know first, and there is no one else who can better convey this information. Frequently, the treating physician may not know with certainty, but a range is acceptable and removes mystery and guesswork by the patient and families.

2. *Physicians should inform patients of how long a procedure will take.* A great physician will assume that the patient knows nothing and will provide clarity, including the amount of time needed to finish a procedure and the anticipated recovery time.

3. *Physicians should tell patients when they will receive information regarding major diagnostic studies or biopsies.* Physicians should leave no ambiguity here and should let the patient and family know when studies will be available and how they will be contacted.

4. *Physicians should inform patients of how they will be informed of routine results.* "No news is good news" is a major patient dissatisfier and is not the platform of a successful clinical operation. Physicians should have a standardized method of informing patients of routine studies. Options can include mailed letters, nurse phone calls, e-mail (secured), or access to the patient's own electronic health record in a password-protected website.

The patient experience and opinion of systems and physicians can hinge on the consistency of staff and physicians keeping patients informed. Physicians are not directly involved in all elements of this component of care, but training physicians on the impact and importance of durations is essential. When physicians are coached and trained on the profound influence of wait times on patient satisfaction, physicians are far more likely to support systemic efforts to keep patients informed.

When physicians see logic and evidence that doing things differently can improve an outcome and that the change effort is within easy, low-lying reach, they will begin to do it themselves and expect it of others. Though coaching physicians will not provide for every element of the patient experience directly, it will create physician influence to change other members of the care team. When physicians step up in the outpatient or emergency room environments and say, "The data is convincing that patients who are kept informed of waits are significantly more satisfied with care. We need to get this done," there exists a compelling physician directive that creates urgency for others. When trained physicians begin to speak up in support of change, there is validation that the change is clinically important, and not just an administrative activity. When physicians round on nursing and ancillary support and request that patients be kept informed, staff will do so. When physicians are running behind and ask patients if they were kept informed of waits, and then provide direct feedback to staff, greater staff accountability and consistency is achieved. Physician training is intended to turn physicians from passive players in a delivery system to captains of teams that work together to improve care and service to patients. Physician influence and input into care operations are drivers of physician satisfaction, and both physician influence and physician satisfaction are served by empowering physicians to drive change.

Coaching physicians on the importance of keeping patients informed is as much about providing physicians with the guidance necessary to improve patient perception as it is about leveraging the physician influence to solidify the training of others.

EXPLANATION

One of the best attendings I ever had gave me great advice as a resident physician. When advising patients, he simply told me to "explain everything." Explanation of medications, treatments, therapies, and follow-ups are key elements of the physician coaching curriculum. When coaching physicians on providing information to patients, there are several key principles to convey:

1. The quality of information patients receive and the understanding they have about the diagnosis and treatment plan can improve adherence to treatment regimens.

2. Physicians do not consistently provide patients with the most fundamental clinical information that can significantly influence medication compliance. A recent study was conducted

regarding physicians' explanations of newly prescribed medications. Twenty-six percent of physicians failed to provide the name of the medication, 13 percent failed to provide the purpose of the medication, 65 percent failed to mention adverse effects, and 66 percent failed to review the duration of treatment.[22] Patient unawareness of basic medication information, mediated through inadequate physician communication, will compromise adherence to treatment regimens.

3. In 2005, Mayo Clinic Proceedings published a study reporting patients' understanding of their diagnosis and medications after discharge from a teaching hospital in Brooklyn, New York. Seventy-two percent were unable to list their discharge medications, and 58 percent were unable to state their discharge diagnosis.[23]

4. Compliance with chronic medical regimens has been estimated to be as low as 30 to 50 percent. Many experts believe that the probability of patient compliance with medications is predicted and driven by the patient's knowledge of his or her diagnosis, the physician-communicated benefit of a medication, and the trust and relationship between the patient and treating physician.

Explaining clinical information to patients is at the core of quality and safety, and training efforts need to be positioned in this way to physicians. Providing training to improve clinical effectiveness is sometimes an easier "sell" to physicians than is training to improve patients' perception of care.

The content of training *"explaining"* is best divided into diagnosis, medications, treatment options, and follow-up care.

DIAGNOSIS: There are components of information that we know patients want when learning of a new diagnosis or condition. Here is what physicians need to explain to patients:

1. **The name of the diagnosis.** Patients want to know what they have. If a physician does not know a definitive diagnosis, then the physician needs to provide a list of possibilities based on presenting symptoms and exam findings. Patients appreciate physicians who convey possibilities when diagnostic uncertainty exists. Equally important, informing and reassuring patients of serious diseases that they *do not* have can be as important as knowing what they *do* have.

2. **Use language the patient can understand.** Medical terminology is acceptable, but it must be followed by a clear and simple explanation of what the terms mean.

3. **The natural history of the stated diagnosis.** Patients want to know what they should expect. Patients will need to know the timing of a therapeutic improvement and when things will get better. Patients appreciate and value this information, even if it may not be what they want to hear. Providing this information to patients can reduce calls back to the office if patients understand an anticipated clinical time course and the natural history of a condition.

4. **Diagnostic testing.** If there is a list of diagnostic possibilities and further information is needed to clarify the diagnosis, physicians should explain this to patients, including what will be involved in the testing procedures. "We need to get a CT scan," means little to patients. Explain the nature of the test, what will be done, and what specifically is being looked for.

5. **Query the patient for his or her understanding.** "Is there any more information you need on your diagnosis?" It is very important to give a patient a specific opportunity to ask questions. Some physicians have used the technique of having patients repeat the information back to the physician to confirm and verify understanding.

6. **Provide written information.** Written information regarding the diagnosis improves patient perception of care. Printed information should include a simple explanation of the condition, self-treatment responsibilities, and return precautions.

A patient's knowledge of his or her diagnosis can lay the foundation for patient partnership, accountability, and responsibility for treatment. A patient's diagnostic ignorance creates treatment indifference and compromises compliance, and can unravel evidence-based treatment plans. It is the patient who most frequently creates the outcome in chronic disease management, not the physician. It is very difficult for patients to invest themselves in treatment plans when they don't have knowledge and understanding of their own diagnosis.

MEDICATIONS: National data has demonstrated that physicians do not consistently provide the most basic of medication information and explanation to patients. In a study assessing discharge patient education, 51 percent of elderly patients discharged from the hospital reported receiving no medication education from the primary treating physician or pharmacist.

How and what the physician says to patients about a medication can heavily impact the probability that the patient will take the medication. When physicians explain medications to patients, the following should be included:

1. The name of the medication.
2. The purpose of the medication. Patient awareness of the therapeutic intent of a medication improves long-term compliance.
3. Potential side effects. When patients are told ahead of time what to look for and what to expect, discontinuation rates decrease.
4. The duration of anticipated treatment. Failure to communicate duration can result in patients "finishing" their medication after the initial 30-day prescription of a new life-long medication.
5. Physicians should explain *why* they selected a particular medication, particularly with asymptomatic diseases like hypertension and diabetes, when the "why" is less clear to patients.
6. A query of patient understanding. Patients are not likely to ask questions unless given a dedicated opportunity to do so. "Is there any more information you need on this medication?" Physicians should give the patient the opportunity to say, "I understand."
7. A query of the patient comfort with the medication and treatment plan. "Are you comfortable with this treatment recommendation?" If patients are uncomfortable with a medication and physicians do not discover this, non-compliance rates will climb. The patient's voice needs to be heard, and his or her opinion and treatment preference solicited. The voices and preferences of patients are foundational to collaboration, patient-centered care, and compliance with medication regimens.

It has been shown that those patients who understand the purpose, potential side effects, duration of therapy, and anticipated outcomes of medications are more likely to take them. Perhaps most predictive of whether a patient will do what a physician recommends is how the patient feels about the physician who recommended the treatment plan. Did the physician seem to care about the patient? Did the physician express interest in the patient's concerns? Did the physician speak to the person or simply pursue the diagnosis? A physician's behavior and conduct with patients can create or dismantle his or her own clinical effectiveness. Extraordinary technical skill means little in the absence of earning patient trust and having influence over what patients do.

TREATMENT OPTIONS: For nearly all conditions, a variety of treatment options exist. Physicians are no longer in a position to mandate treatment for patients. Responsibility for treatment decisions is now shared. Physicians should recommend and advise based on medical evidence and experience, but it is the patient who makes the final decision. The physician's ability to review treatment options is a key element of building an effective, collaborative partnership to achieve therapeutic outcomes. Coaching physicians should include the following elements:

1. If several reasonable treatment options exist, review those with patients. Physicians should assume that patients have researched their own condition and will have a vague, sometimes misguided, sense of what is available. A physician who fails to cover known treatment options can undermine patient confidence.

2. Which treatment is selected should be based on two key factors:

    a. The patient preference: Physicians should ask the patient for his or her wishes in terms of treatment options as a sincere effort to find out what the patient wants. Soliciting patients' input is the cornerstone of collaboration and shared decision making.
    b. The physician recommendation: Physicians should convey their recommendation based on evidence. If physicians

> have earned the trust of patients, it is likely that the physician recommendation will heavily impact patient decision making. Patient-centered care should never be confused with patients doing whatever they want. Patients want a physician who can make a clear and confident recommendation based on his or her expertise.

FOLLOW-UP CARE: When patients finish an encounter with a physician in any clinical environment, they should be made aware of what will be happening next. Patients should be given clear verbal and written directions on follow-up issues, including the following:

1. Appointments: If patients are discharged from the hospital, the timing of follow-up should be included in all discharge documents. Patients should know with whom they are to follow up and the purpose of every hospital discharge follow-up visit. Likewise, in an outpatient environment, patients should have clarity and understanding of when and with whom they are to follow up. When patients do not have follow-up information, a physician and the system run the risk of a patient slipping through the cracks. When patients know the purpose and intentions of follow-up, they become more involved and engaged in their own care plan, and follow-up compliance is improved.

2. Return precautions: Patients should be given clear, documented guidelines for clinical indications for return. This communication is important for patient safety as well as physician and hospital litigation protection.

THANK YOU

The *thank you* of AIDET is about the closure of the encounter and the final, lasting impression the patient leaves with. As with the first impression, the last impression makes a notable imprint on patients.

Key elements in training physicians in "thank you" and visit closure:

1. Physicians who take a pause to thank patients for seeking care with them will surprise and delight patients. This should never be forced or artificial, but a genuine expression of appreciation.
2. What physicians say in their last words is what patients leave with. "I am glad you came in today; I know we can help." This statement from physicians validates the patient's concern as important. If a clinical concern is important to a patient, it IS important, no matter how "trivial" it may seem to physicians. The physician who at any time belittles or disregards a patient's concern will lose that patient forever. Additionally, this closing statement provides for optimism and an encouraging expectation, which is exactly what patients want from a physician. Never misrepresent medical facts, but never miss the opportunity to communicate hope.
3. Recognize patients for work done. Patients who exercise to lose weight, who work hard to achieve glycemic control, and who quit smoking after years of counsel should be specifically and deliberately recognized by physicians. Physician acknowledgment of specific behaviors will propagate behaviors. A physician who says, "Your commitment and hard work are really making a difference—you are really doing a fantastic job. Keep up the good work." How does this close compare to that of the physician who does not notice, recognize, or acknowledge patient efforts? Recognizing, acknowledging, and thanking patients take almost no time and can solidify the close of a clinical encounter.

TRAINING PHYSICIANS IN ELECTRONIC RECORD USE

Many systems intend to use or have already rolled out electronic health records (EHR). The EHR represents a new and significant set of challenges and can fundamentally change the patient experience. If this element of care is not done properly, patients can leave a clinical encounter feeling disregarded, ignored, and frustrated with the invasion of the computer into the exam room.

When electronic records are activated, training physicians is an important element to a successful rollout. The EHR should improve the patient experience, as patients desire physicians and systems to be "connected" with seamless communication over time and locations. Electronic records afford the opportunity for patients to view results online, to gain access to drug and disease information, to request medication refills, and to receive electronic alerts regarding their own health maintenance reminders. Most importantly, the EHR, properly positioned, allows patients to become engaged in their own medical records. The realization of benefits for an EHR will depend on physicians doing it "right."

Key trainable tactics to improve the patient experience with an electronic health record include:

- The electronic record use should not be trained as an electronic version of a paper chart, but as a unique opportunity to include patients and to share information.
- Computers should be physically positioned to allow patients to see the record if they so choose. The computer should draw the patient into the encounter instead of pulling the physician away from the patient.
- Demonstrate to patients the capabilities of the electronic record with trending results, information access, disease management, and electronic prescribing. A 30-second "road test" can demonstrate to patients the capabilities of a new system.

- Physicians must keep the patient as the focal point of an encounter. If physicians fail to engage and connect with patients in exchange for a quick "log-in" to the EHR, patients are likely to view the computer as an intrusion that deflects the physician's attention away from them.
- If data entry is necessary during the clinical encounter, physicians should simply explain what they are doing, and ask if it is okay.

"As you tell me about your symptoms, I am going to enter this information into the computer as part of your medical record. I want to make sure that is okay with you. Let me show you what I am doing."

- Simple disclosure, recognition, and permission to enter data can circumvent patient perception that the computer has taken the focus off the patient. Conversely, if physicians fail to explain activities up-front, patients will wonder, "What is this doctor doing?" The uninformed, disregarded patient is the patient who will most assuredly leave frustrated.
- Patient information generated from many EHRs can leave important final impressions for patients. Information on medications, diagnosis, self-treatment options, return precautions, contact information, and follow-up care are important communications that the electronic record can consistently generate. Key words are important in leveraging information generated by the electronic record to improve patient communication. A stack of papers handed to a discharged patient does little to improve quality, safety, or the patient experience. Key words are phrases that provoke a

predictable positive impression and can be used by physicians or nurses to enhance information transfer.

- o Key words that can improve communication and the patient's perception of care include the following:
    - *To keep you informed* about your discharge medications and diagnosis…
    - We *care about you* and about how you are doing after your discharge, and we want to make sure that you get your follow-up care…
    - We want to be sure that we *keep you comfortable* and manage your pain well…
    - We want to make sure that we answer all of your questions and that you *understand your discharge instructions…*
- The key to driving the patient experience in systems using the EHR is to position the electronic record positively. If physicians are frustrated with the electronic record, do not share that private information with patients. Nobody wins when physicians mock the EHR in the presence of patients.

A physician champion should be tasked with integrating physician EHR communication training with the AIDET curriculum. For those organizations that have made a commitment to electronic records, the importance of physicians' effective use of technology in the exam room must be conveyed in training. A successful rollout of an EHR is about institutionalizing how it is used by those caring for patients. Simple guidance can help physicians realize the benefits of technology at the bedside to improve patient care. In time, the EHR will become an indispensable component of care, a way to mine data, a method to track quality, a means to communicate electronically, and a way to create a shared record to establish active patient involvement in patients' own care.

SUMMARY OF PHYSICIAN TRAINING

AIDET changes healthcare delivery and is a foundation to build systemwide behavioral consistency, marketplace reputation, and differentiation. Systems are only as good as how they perform all of the time. Like any other strategy, AIDET is only as effective as its implementation. AIDET training can be done as a singular training event for physicians, but the elements of AIDET will need to be reminded and prompted by physician champions to sustain change. For physicians, implementation and uptake of AIDET is impacted and predicted not only by the effectiveness of AIDET physician training, but by the execution of Stages 1 through 4 that precede physician training. AIDET is an investment in physicians to make them more successful and a reflection of the value and importance of the physician workforce as a precious system asset. When this sentiment is sensed by physicians and physicians feel that the system has brought them value in training, receptiveness to a shared mission is created.

I recently coached Methodist Hospital System in San Antonio. After the session, I was reading physician comments and encountered one that read, "Thank you, Methodist, for helping me be a better physician. This is what I want healthcare to be." Training delivers evidence-based behaviors that will improve care to patients, but more importantly, investment in physicians will create loyalty to work together to make healthcare what it should be. Training that is useful, practical, and makes physicians better is a powerful physician engagement and alignment strategy. Physicians will do for the system what system leaders have done for physicians.

Success will come to a system when AIDET is done by everyone, all of the time. Sustainable physician behavioral change is a complex process that requires more than isolated coaching and training as a singular, siloed event. Jumping directly to physician AIDET training without the staged assembly of vision, goals, leadership, accountability, administrative responsiveness, and physician leader visibility will blunt the transformational impact that AIDET implementation should have.

Key Learnings for Stage 5, "Training Physicians":

1. Important components of "Training Physicians" include the following:
   a. If AIDET is not demonstrated by physicians, then the impact of AIDET training for the rest of the healthcare team is lessened.
   b. AIDET training improves patient satisfaction.
   c. AIDET aligns physician behaviors with an organizational commitment to improve care for patients.
   d. AIDET provides communication skills to physicians that position them to be more successful.
   e. A system that invests in and exerts efforts to improve physicians' care for patients can create loyalty to the system and its leaders.
2. The sequence of physician training is important. Isolated "behavioral training" rarely changes behaviors on a long-term basis.
3. The sequence will include:
   a. Creating physician buy-in.
   b. Creating an internal "burning platform" that mandates change.
   c. Providing AIDET training.
4. Physician training should be done by physicians, preferably internal physician champions.
5. The content of AIDET will need to be repeated to maintain consistency of behaviors.
6. Training physicians on how to use the EHR to improve patient communication is an important element of an EHR rollout.

STAGE 6:
Physician Measurement and Balanced Scorecards

"Words are words, explanations are explanations, promises are promises. Only performance is reality."

—Harold Geneen

Physicians who are effectively trained in AIDET and who practice in a system that possesses clear vision and goals as well as collaborative, responsive leadership will enroll most physicians to support the organizational mission. Is this enough to predictably and reliably change physician behavior? Stages 1 through 5 can initiate and grow physician participation in system change, but there are other key components to creating consistent, sustainable physician effort and performance improvement. The application of measuring and reporting individual physician performance using balanced scorecards is a key stage to drive and intensify physician effort to achieve physician-supported system goals.

Leaders will frequently ask, "What is the one thing that changes physician behavior the most?" It is, without question, the measurement and reporting of physician performance compared to peers on measures physicians care about. Initial traction for physician change can be challenging in the absence of physician performance data. Physician performance measurement illuminates current and specific performance and provides the logic behind change efforts. Measurement is the tracking device to determine what is working and provides a means to identify those who struggle. Measurement is the differentiator between the good and the great, the reality check and the counterpunch to the "if it's not broken, don't fix it" organizational epitaph. Consider measurement of performance to be the fuel for the physician engagement pathway and a necessity for meaningful behavioral change.

Physicians are very sensitive to how they compare to colleagues on measures of professional performance. Tracking, reporting, and benchmarking door to doc times by individual physician reduces door to doc times and improves patient flow. When a physician receives a performance report that reveals he is seeing 1.6 patients per hour (the lowest average in the emergency department), compared to a peer average of 2.6, that physician becomes attentive to improving measured performance. When the "patients seen per hour" data set becomes transparent, posted in the physician lounge, attention and the drive to improve become even more compelling. Without awareness of performance data, would a physician seeing 1.6 patients per hour be driven or inspired to change? Getting physicians out of the old way of doing things is hard enough. Without performance measurement as an argument for change, change may never begin.

Physician change initiation is complex and relies on accurate and realistic physician performance reflection. The problem with this change process is that physicians tend to have a fairly high opinion of what they do and how they do things. I was recently with a group of 80 physicians in northern California. I asked this group of physicians how many of them thought they were "above average" in managing the composite of diabetes care. Every physician in the room raised his or her hand. I told them that it was *not* possible that every physician in the room was above average. Physician self-assessment, in the absence of objective performance measurement, almost always overestimates reality. If physicians are "of the opinion" that they are doing things well, why in the world should they change? Measurement and performance reporting are the change initiators. The presence of a clear record demonstrating where a physician stands relative to benchmarks makes the argument for change more difficult for physicians to overrun.

Though the application of measurement can be a strong driver of physician change, it also has the potential to create physician protest and opposition. This stage must be done cautiously, with all foundational stages in place. Stages 1 through 5 will position a system performance culture with clear and visible goals, in which individual physician measurement, performance, and accountability will be seen as a logical organizational progression. Effective physician leadership will position measurement as verification of performance for a renewed outcomes-driven, evidence-based system. The relationships with the medical staff established in Stage 3 will be needed to support the measurement stage. If there is distrust, animosity, or significant "issues" between leadership and physicians, then measuring and reporting physician performance will come under intense heat, protest, and rejection from physicians.

Even with solid physician relations, physician performance measurement is likely to draw animated discussion among physicians, and will invariably stir opinion and commentary as comparative performance measures are reported. This focus, interest, and attention on physician performance measures is exactly why measurement has a potentially significant impact on physician behavior and why it will serve as a key accelerator to implementation of service and quality initiatives.

The following represents core principles in the effective application of measurement to improve physician efforts and align behaviors.

WHICH PHYSICIANS CAN BE "MEASURED"?

The application of physician performance measurement applies principally to employed or contracted physicians. Individual physician scorecards on service and quality measures will be more challenging to collect and report for the private affiliated physicians in a hospital system. It is important for health system leaders to remember several facts regarding the tracking and reporting of physician performance to the seemingly elusive affiliated staff members:

- The evolution of hospitalists as the most rapidly growing specialty will drive the "employed/contracted" model.
- Affiliated physicians are taking care of smaller portions of inpatient admissions as hospitalists assume a greater patient load.
- Larger multispecialty groups are growing and providing further employed opportunities for physicians as overhead costs limit private practice growth.
- Even if a system does not employ hospitalists, in most cases 20 percent of affiliated medical staff members will perform 80 percent of the inpatient work. This high volume group should be the initial focus of engagement and performance measurement reporting efforts.

The application of physician measurement will not apply to every system, but can be useful to many. Measurement and scorecards can be effectively applied to employed or contracted physicians in the inpatient, outpatient, urgent care, and emergency room environments.

PRINCIPLES OF REPORTING PERFORMANCE TO PHYSICIANS

The method of performance communication to physicians and how it is perceived is as important as the measurements themselves. If this step is done improperly, it will, at best, have little impact on physician effort and behavior. At worst, improperly applied measurement of physicians can unravel the engagement efforts that the system has worked so hard to achieve in Stages 1 through 5.

Key elements in effectively communicating measurement performance to physicians include the following:

- Performance measures must be consistent with the system vision and goals that have been clearly communicated by leadership in Stage 1. The renewed system vision is now about a performance culture and executing superior, measurable outcomes. Physicians will respect this platform, and measuring and reporting performance will make sense in this context.
- Physician "group" performance reporting rarely impacts individual behaviors. Individual physician performance reporting, in line with system goals, will create effort and change. When a group of hospitalists gets a report of general "physician" 30-day readmit rates, those measures draw a look. When 30-day readmit rates are transparently reported by individual physicians, this will draw intense focus and impact clinical behavior.
- Goal selection, as articulated in Stage 1, will have been created with heavy physician input and should be communicated to medical staff as such. Goals that appear to be administrative or regulatory are a much tougher sell to physicians. Physician leadership visibility, communication, and support of goals will be key here.

- When system goals are based on medical evidence, are created with physician input, and are beneficial to physicians and patients, physician support for goals is more likely. When physicians commit to supporting goals, the "case" for measurement and verification of performance is much stronger and less likely to be protested by the medical staff.

USING MEASUREMENT TO CHANGE BEHAVIORS

The purpose of measurement is never to scold, embarrass, or humiliate physicians. The purpose and spirit of measurement is to improve. Individual knowledge and awareness of where one stands relative to others and relative to an articulated goal are the core principles of measurement application to drive effort and align behavior.

Imagine if we were to measure and report individual physician "hand washing" on a clinical unit, and how frequently physicians comply with CDC standards of washing their hands before and after every patient contact. From this measurement data we create a comparative rank list of physicians from top to bottom by frequency of hand washing. Then we take that comparative measurement data set and post it on the community board for everyone to see. What would the process of measuring and reporting hand washing frequency do to the probability of physicians washing their hands? Who wants to be at the bottom of that data set? Reporting of hand washing has nothing to do with training physicians to wash their hands. Measurement and the reporting of performance in a comparative database uses illumination and awareness of data to intensify efforts to achieve measured outcomes.

When reporting physician performance measures, one must walk the fine line between establishing worthy goals that create effort and incentive to achieve versus engaging in performance reporting that splinters trust and damages the relationship between administration and physicians.

Here are important principles in optimizing the impact of physician measurement:

- System goals and individual physician goals should "match." Physician awareness of system goals (Stage 1) reduces uncertainty and creates a logical alignment of physician efforts consistent with worthy, physician-selected organizational goals.
- Absolute "raw" physician performance measure reporting does little to impact physician effort in contrast to comparative performance reporting. Measurement of physicians' performance compared to peers is far more likely to create interest, attention, and effort. When physicians see that they have "left without being seen" (LWBS) in the emergency room of 3.8 percent, it means little and has marginal influence on physician behavior. When physicians see 3.8 percent LWBS in the context of a comparative report with a physician peer average of 1.2 percent, the same measure can draw attention, stir emotion, and change behavior.
- The ultimate application of comparative measurement is full transparency of performance measures. Achieving full transparency for physician performance is a slow, progressive process that can take several years. It is recommended to initiate blind comparative measurements in which a physician can see his or her individual performance relative to blinded colleagues. As physicians become comfortable with comparative reporting, results are progressively unblinded, beginning with small departments and moving toward full staff transparency.
- Protest will arise during the pathway to transparency. It is very important for physician leaders to go slow and to provide ongoing communication and feedback regarding collective physician performance, system goals, and the direct linkage between the two. If physicians fall out on performance measures, the system and leadership must respond. The voice of

> leaders to struggling physicians is not, "You are not doing well enough; do it better!" In fact, the nature of intervention is to help and assist, and to do whatever it takes to help physicians improve. The physician champions will be trained in this role, particularly on patient satisfaction measures. Sitting idle and doing nothing when a physician is repeatedly below standards is unfair to patients, the system, and the physician.

Comparative, transparent measurement reporting of physician performance, when coupled with AIDET training and vision-driven leadership, will create progressive physician alignment towards system goals and organizational culture.

Within the Sharp Rees-Stealy Medical Group, a nearly 400-physician multi-specialty practice, quality performance measures are reported with full transparency. When physicians' performance measures and clinical markers are visible to colleagues, this changes physician focus to achieve reported performance. I have attended meetings in which individual physician clinical markers are placed on PowerPoint for all physicians to see. Physicians will do everything in their power to improve comparative, transparent performance. Prior to individual physician measurement and reporting, there were few means by which to differentiate those at the top of clinical and service measures from those at the bottom. In the absence of meaningful feedback, our physicians simply did what they always did, with little attention or effort toward improvement. This was not done out of laziness or indifference; they were simply unaware. Without measurement, knowledge of performance, and transparency of measures, what drives one to move and do things differently?

The Sharp Rees-Stealy Medical Group has now been ranked the number one system in the state of California for three consecutive years in clinical quality and the patient experience.[24] Transparent measurement reporting was a foundational catalyst to physician alignment and the effort to achieve our success.

PHYSICIAN PERFORMANCE MEASURES

Deciding what to measure for physician performance comes down to determining what the physicians will pursue and what the system will achieve. "What gets measured gets done" makes the selection of performance markers for the physician scorecard a very important organizational decision. In selecting physician performance measures, the focus should be on creating a balanced, "pillar-based" approach designed to foster and align key physician behaviors to achieve system goals.

When deciding what to place as measures for a physician performance scorecard, it is key to use system goals as the backbone. If physicians achieve individual clinical and service goals, so too will the system. If the physician's performance scorecard is heavily weighted on quality measures, that is what the system will achieve. If a scorecard has no representation for patient satisfaction, consistent physician delivery of service will be lessened. If scorecards place generic utilization for medications, that area will improve. If a system wants to drive physician meeting attendance, designate this as a performance measure.

Important pillar-based physician performance measures can include:

1. **Quality:** Clinical quality measure performance is commonplace now, and should continue to be an important component in assessing and reporting physician performance. Quality measures can include adoption of evidence-based guidelines, clinical markers for disease management, core measures, and outcomes that reflect physician clinical performance.

2. **Service:** Patient satisfaction is a key indicator of physician performance assessment and should be included on all balanced scorecards. Assessing patient satisfaction is intended to reflect

the physician interaction with patients and its impact on patient loyalty, listening, clarity of communication, involving patients in healthcare decisions, and the likelihood of a patient recommending a physician to others.

3. **Finance:** When applying physician performance assessment methods in the recent past, revenue production was often the sole or dominant measure. "Eat what you kill" was a pervasive mantra. When physicians are assessed solely on productivity, there is less attention, drive, and motivation for other key competencies that make for exceptional physicians, successful systems, and balanced performance. Though financial productivity is important and at the core of practice success, it must be part of other pillar performance measures and not more, or less, important.

4. **People:** How physicians treat staff and fellow colleagues can be as important as how they treat patients. Even a clinically excellent physician with a stellar reputation in the community among patients can unravel a site or department by how he or she treats nursing staff and physician colleagues. Nurses' perception of physicians and fellow physicians' opinions of each other as a reported performance measure can align physicians to "do the right thing." The spirit of cooperation and collaboration should be a measurable outcome for physician performance. Physicians care deeply about physician colleague and nurse opinion. The process of collecting nurse and colleague observations is a measure of teamwork. Providing feedback to physicians regarding what others see can change what physicians do.

5. **Growth:** Many will say that patient satisfaction is simply a precursor for the most important patient experience measure: the loyalty of the patients seen by physicians. A physician's

ability to generate referrals to him or herself and to the system is a key indicator of physician performance. Even if the physician performs well by all other pillar measures, but does not bring growth and word of mouth referrals, practice and system success will be limited.

Clinical excellence, patient satisfaction and loyalty, financial productivity, and the respectful, collaborative treatment of fellow physicians and staff members is the definition of a high-performing physician today. There is not a single physician pillar measure that can be overlooked or disregarded. To assure and verify execution of these critical competencies, a balanced, comparative physician scorecard must be created. Balanced performance feedback will lay the foundation for assessing, reporting, reflecting, and improving actions and behaviors that will create physician and system performance across pillars.

An outline for performance indicators is presented to provide options on what to select for physician scorecards. These will be presented by healthcare environment including outpatient, inpatient, and emergency room performance indicators. Specialty markers are not included in this option list, but are available at cms.hhs.gov/PQRI. This PDF document contains the complete specifications for the 119 measures that make up the 2008 Physician Quality Reporting Initiative (PQRI).

OUTPATIENT PHYSICIAN PERFORMANCE MEASURES

OUTPATIENT QUALITY MEASURES: Which performance indicators an organization selects depends on the system goals that are in place. It is recommended to survey the local regulatory environment when determining which measures should be pursued. As Pay for Performance evolves and expands, it is logical to select system goals that are consistent with local performance benchmarks. The number of goals placed under the quality pillar will be an individual system decision, but can climb as high as 12. Having more than 12 goals tends to diminish impact and create measurement dilution.

Outpatient quality measures:

1. Patients with type I/II Diabetes (DM) with hga1c greater than 9.0 (poor control)
2. Patients with DM with LDL <100
3. Patients with DM with annual urinary micro-albumin assessment
4. Patients with DM with annual monofilament
5. Patients with DM and HTN on ACE/ARB
6. Patients with type I/II with hga1c of <7.0
7. Patients with all of the diabetes composite care and control elements
8. Patients with chronic kidney disease on ACE/ARB
9. ASA use in patients with CAD
10. ASA/ACE and beta blocker use in patients with CAD and CHF
11. Blood pressure less than 140/90 in patients with HTN
12. Blood pressure less than 130/80 in patients with DM
13. Screening mammography per guidelines
14. Colorectal cancer screening per guidelines
15. Cervical cancer screening per guidelines
16. Inquiry regarding tobacco use
17. Counseling regarding smoking cessation
18. Influenza vaccination for patients >50 or high risk
19. Pneumonia vaccination for patients >65
20. Screening for osteoporosis in women >65
21. Avoidance of lumbar x-rays for uncomplicated lower back pain
22. Avoidance of antibiotics in patients with uncomplicated acute bronchitis
23. Asthma (mild, moderate, or severe persistent) diagnosis with controller medication
24. Depression screening for patients with chronic illnesses

25. COPD patients with spirometry done
26. COPD patients with FEV, 70 percent predicted on bronchodilator therapy
27. Documentation of an Advanced Directive

OUTPATIENT SERVICE MEASURES: Many larger healthcare systems will pay outside vendors to assess the patient experience through mail or phone surveys. These results can easily be imported and "uploaded" into an individual physician scorecard. When utilizing outside vendors, organizations will have the ability to compare performance to a national comparative database, as well as to save the administrative work required to conduct independent, internal patient surveys. The key to effectively reporting service performance to physicians is the ability to provide specific patient feedback and to use measurement to evaluate what the physician did and didn't do. The patient perception *is* the physician reality, regardless of what the physician *thinks* he or she did. Reporting physician behaviors from the patient perspective is vital as a performance indicator and as a learning instrument. Feedback should be specific enough to translate to actionable physician coaching and specific performance improvement.

Depending on the question format, responses can vary by frequency of behaviors (always, usually, sometimes, and never) or by grade (one through five, or very good, good, fair, poor, very poor.) The progression toward frequency reporting in standardized patient experience measures is noteworthy. As physician and system performance is reported using frequency analysis (always, usually, sometimes, and never), physicians will get "credit" only for an *always* response. Physicians and organizations measuring the patient experience with a frequency analysis tool will get no credit for doing something most of the time.

Common patient questions can include the following:

Frequency assessment (never, sometimes, usually, always)

1. How often did this physician explain things in a way you could understand?
2. How often did this physician spend enough time with you?
3. How often did this physician listen carefully to your concerns?
4. How often did this physician know important information about your health history?
5. How often did this physician include you in healthcare decisions?
6. How often were you seen within 15 minutes of your appointment?
7. How often did this physician provide you with information regarding follow-up care?
8. When you called this physician during regular office hours, how often did you get an answer to your question the same day?
9. When you had a blood test or x-ray, how often did the physician's office contact you regarding test results?

Scaled assessment (1-5/ very poor, poor, fair, good, very good)

10. How would you rate your physician's friendliness? (1-5)
11. Were you given adequate explanation of your medical condition? (1-5)
12. Did your physician show concerns for your questions? (1-5)
13. How well were you included in decisions regarding your health? (1-5)
14. Were you given adequate information about medications? (1-5)
15. Were you given clear information regarding follow-up care? (1-5)
16. Did your physician spend adequate time with you? (1-5)
17. How would you rate this physician overall? (1-5)
18. Would you recommend this physician to family and friends? (1-5)

The dashboard of patient satisfaction should be presented and communicated so that it is clear in regard to physician strengths and weaknesses, as well as what needs to be done in order to improve. Individual physician coaching intervention should use this specific performance data as the template for intervention tactics.

OUTPATIENT PEOPLE MEASURES: There are two important elements in measuring physician performance under the people ("teamwork") pillar. These performance measures include physician interaction and communication with physician colleagues and with nursing staff. The underlying purpose of *all* measurement is improvement and feedback to help physicians identify what they do well and what needs to change. In my coaching experience, measuring and reporting peer and staff observations of physician behavior draws more focus than all other measures.

I recently worked with a system that was having difficulty with physicians' treatment of nurses on an inpatient unit. Physician leaders, who were well aware of these issues, approved a pilot program in which nurses on that unit could anonymously review physician behaviors. The data was collected to create an honest assessment of the nurses' work experience with physicians, and their observations were reported back to physicians. Six months after the initiative began, I spoke with the charge nurse who had led this project and asked if the feedback from nurses to physicians changed physicians' behavior. She said to me, with a big smile on her face, "They have turned into a group of angels." Physicians had little awareness of or insight into their own behavior and its impact on the work experience for nurses. Physicians *cannot change* if they are unaware of what they are doing. For physicians to do things differently, this message must be delivered directly to them. The physicians on this unit didn't realize that they were intimidating. They didn't know that nurses saw them as "moody" and unpredictable. They didn't realize that they would walk away from a nurse halfway through a question until there was clear, honest, and deliberate feedback given in the spirit of making physician/nurse relationships better.

Physicians care deeply about nurse and colleague opinions of them, and will frequently increase their effort and correct their behaviors when the realities of day-to-day interactions are respectfully communicated.

NURSE REVIEW OF PHYSICIAN INTERACTIONS: These are question sets that nurses can answer about outpatient physician interactions.

Figure 6.1

NURSE FEEDBACK ON PHYSICIAN INTERACTIONS SURVEY SAMPLE

Nurse Feedback Practice

In order to continually improve quality of care, the physicians of (Name) Medical Group request your assistance in assessing physician performance. Please answer the following questionnaire in an honest and thoughtful manner. The responses will be collated and summarized for each physician in confidence and used as feedback to try to improve patient care and interaction with office staff.

As a member of the office team, I am a:

____ Nurse ____Medical Assistant ____Tech ____Admin Assistant ____Other

Physician:	
Reviewer:	
Date:	

Scale:

5 - Strongly agree / Always performs
4 - Agree / Performs on most occasions
3 - Fair / Inconsistently performs
2 - Disagree / Usually does not perform
1 - Strongly disagree / Does not perform
N/A - Not in significant contact with this physician

Sees and treats patients in a timely manner	1	2	3	4	5	N/A
Stays on schedule and prioritizes well	1	2	3	4	5	N/A
Arrives on time and communicates whereabouts when leaving	1	2	3	4	5	N/A
Treats staff in a professional and courteous manner	1	2	3	4	5	N/A
Effectively communicates to staff and is easily approachable with questions	1	2	3	4	5	N/A
Appreciates and recognizes staff for their efforts	1	2	3	4	5	N/A
Writes legibly and completes documentation in a timely manner	1	2	3	4	5	N/A
Shows caring and concern for patients/their families	1	2	3	4	5	N/A
Overall rating of the total care of patients by this physician	1	2	3	4	5	N/A
Overall rating of the ease of working with this physician	1	2	3	4	5	N/A

Total Score ________________

Average Score ________________

Please comment regarding working with this physician. Please provide positive work experiences as well as concerns or problems.

Comments

The dynamic between physicians and nursing staff is one of the most important relationships within a care delivery system. Patient safety, clinical outcomes, staff turnover, and workplace culture are at stake. The impact of abusive physician behaviors toward nurses makes it an imperative physician performance measure. Historically, nurses will use this as an instrument to rave about the physicians they work with. Conversely, if there is physician conduct that is disrespectful and abusive toward staff, this performance measure will find, document, and quantify it. Leadership's ability to intervene on sure footing when difficult and abusive behaviors arise depends on having staff review measurement data to support the stories of disrespectful behaviors.

PEER REVIEW: Peer review is a measurement tool to assess physician-to-physician interaction and communication. The physician clinical work experience and perception of a system is heavily influenced by the relationship a physician has with colleagues. Is physician interaction respectful, collegial, and cooperative, and do physicians work hard together to do the right thing for patients? Or does there exist an isolated, distant, siloed physician workforce in which there is little interaction, little support, and even abusive interactions that can ruin the clinical work experience and threaten patient safety? Collaborative, respectful communication between physicians is embedded in the culture of high-performing organizations, and should be a part of physician orientation, training, and systemwide behavioral standards. To ensure execution and verification of physician-to-physician conduct, measurement, assessment, and documentation of these behaviors should be deployed.

If you have a gastroenterologist who screams at ER physicians every time they call for a gastrointestinal bleed, is there a measurement tool to objectively assess and document this behavior? The spirit of peer review is to observe, measure, and provide feedback for physician behaviors that can support or undermine an organizational culture.

Typically, physicians who work in direct contact with or who give or receive referrals from another physician will fill out a colleague's peer review on an annual basis. Here is an example of a Physician Peer Review template.

Figure 6.2

PHYSICIAN PEER REVIEW SURVEY SAMPLE

Physician Peer Review

Physician interaction and conduct are major determinants in the well-being of our group and the patients we take care of. Please evaluate your physician colleague in a thoughtful and honest manner. Results will be collated and reported to physicians in confidence and used as feedback for performance improvement.

Physician:	
Reviewer:	
Date:	

Scale:

5 - Strongly agree / Always performs
4 - Agree / Performs on most occasions
3 - Fair / Inconsistently performs / Average
2 - Below average / Usually does not perform
1 - Poor / Never performs / Needs major improvement
N/A - Not in significant contact with this physician

Answers pages and calls promptly	1	2	3	4	5	N/A
Treats physician colleagues respectfully	1	2	3	4	5	N/A
Arrives to clinic on time	1	2	3	4	5	N/A
Effectively communicates with staff and is approachable with questions	1	2	3	4	5	N/A
Is willing to help colleagues when needed	1	2	3	4	5	N/A
Shows caring/concern for patients and families	1	2	3	4	5	N/A
Participates/supports QI efforts	1	2	3	4	5	N/A
Demonstrates appropriate clinical management	1	2	3	4	5	N/A
Would recommend to friends and family	1	2	3	4	5	N/A
Overall rating of physician	1	2	3	4	5	N/A

Total Score ________________

Average Score ________________

Please comment on your physician colleague regarding your experience working with this physician. Please specify positive experiences as well as concerns or problems.

Comments

ADDITIONAL PEOPLE PILLAR PHYSICIAN MEASURES: Though physician conduct towards staff and colleagues is vital for the cultivation of the culture and character of a system, other physician behaviors are important in driving physician involvement and participation in organizational change. The process of getting physicians involved is a habitual challenge, and can leave physician and administrative leaders frustrated with poor physician turnouts and participation. Applying the measurement process to other physician engagement measures can improve physician involvement and participation in important operational issues.

Other people performance measures that can impact important physician actions include the following:

1. **Physician meeting attendance:** It is difficult to convey vision, goals, and strategies if physicians do not participate in or attend meetings. Tracking and reporting attendance, creating expectations, and incentivizing attendance can change physician presence and participation. For example, in our organization those physicians who attend 50 percent of meetings throughout the year receive a small bonus at year's end. Our meeting attendance is excellent.
2. **Physician participation in committees or initiatives:** Employed or contracted physicians can have physician participation in committees or initiatives as a measure of physician involvement in system efforts. Offering small financial incentives for physicians who "meet" participation goals can shift the balance for physicians on the fence and prompt them to get involved.

Tracking attendance and conveying expectations for meeting attendance and committee participation increases the likelihood that physicians will get involved. Offering small amounts of incentive money for expectation performance can make a big difference.

OUTPATIENT GROWTH MEASURES: Two of the most important components of system and physician success are keeping patients and growing market share. Do patients stay when they arrive? Is loyalty established? Do patients "promote" and recommend a physician they have seen? These are all aspirations of physicians and important reflections of physician performance. If there is no data measurement stream, how does one know who is doing what and where resources that are intended to help may be needed? Is anyone in a system aware of physicians who lose patients after the first encounter?

Driving growth is the ultimate and final dividend of system and physician performance improvement. Patient loyalty happens when relationships are built and when patients *know* that the physician and the entire organization truly care about them. Patient loyalty is what the system and the physicians must have in order to preserve revenue streams and to meet operating expenses. Measurement and reporting of physician *growth* is verification that efforts are working and are a direct and quantitative reflection of patient loyalty.

Physician Growth Measures:

1. **Patient transfer rates away from a practice:** In many systems that track patients assigned to a primary care physician, transfer rates are a trackable performance measure. Physicians who lose patients through transfers away from their practice at a significantly higher rate than peers would never be identified in the absence of measurement. Similar to low patient satisfaction, high transfer rates should be a coaching intervention criterion for physicians.
2. **Likelihood of recommending a physician:** This is a common question patients are asked on most patient satisfaction surveys. Many believe that this is the single most important question a patient can answer in order to reflect the patient's loyalty to a physician and his or her global satisfaction with care. In fact,

some systems will use this question alone to assess the patient experience delivered by physicians.

INPATIENT PHYSICIAN PERFORMANCE MEASURES

Measuring, reporting, and providing feedback as a means to change physician clinical effort applies similarly to the inpatient, outpatient, or emergency room settings. What is measured and reported is different according to the clinical environment. The specific performance measures that are selected and reported to physicians are a leadership decision and are based on organizational goals that the organization wants to achieve.

INPATIENT QUALITY MEASURES: Physician quality measures most frequently include CMS core measures. These are national benchmarks with significant evidence backing them. Physician inpatient quality measure options are included for reference.

Acute MI Measures:

1. Aspirin prescribed at discharge
2. ACE or ARB for left ventricular dysfunction with ejection fractions less than 40 percent
3. Adult smoking cessation documentation
4. Beta blocker at discharge
5. LDL cholesterol assessment
6. Statin prescribed at discharge

Congestive Heart Failure Measures:

1. Complete discharge education for CHF patients (activity level, diet, discharge medications, follow-up appointment, weight monitoring, and instructions when symptoms worsen)
2. Evaluation of left ventricular function during hospital stay for CHF

3. ACE or ARB for CHF patients with ejection fractions less than 40 percent
4. Smoking cessation counseling documentation in CHF patients

Pneumonia Measures:

1. Oxygen level assessment in patients with pneumonia
2. Pneumonia patients age 65 and older, who were screened for pneumococcal vaccine status and were administered the vaccine prior to discharge, if indicated
3. Adult smoking cessation counseling
4. Time from arrival with a diagnosis of pneumonia to the administration of the first dose of antibiotic
5. Appropriate antibiotic selection for community-acquired pneumonia based on Pneumonia Antibiotic Consensus Recommendations
6. Patients over age 50 who were screened for influenza vaccine status and were administered the vaccine, if appropriate

Surgical Care Measures:

1. Prophylactic antibiotic received within one hour of surgical incision
2. Timely discontinuation of prophylactic antibiotic post-operatively per protocols
3. Surgical patients with appropriate hair removal using clippers
4. Post-operative cardiac patients with blood glucose levels of less than 200 on post-op days one and two
5. Colorectal surgery patients who achieve normothermia within 15 minutes after leaving the operating room
6. Surgery patients on beta blockers pre-operatively who received a beta-blocker during the peri-operative period
7. Surgery patients with recommended venous thromboembolism prophylaxis ordered

Stroke Care Measures:

1. Deep vein prophylaxis for patients with ischemic or hemorrhagic stroke by hospital day two
2. Anti-coagulation use in patients with atrial fibrillation and stroke
3. Anti-platelet agent in stroke patients
4. Dysphagia screening in stroke patients
5. Physical therapy assessment in stroke patients

Overall Quality Measures:

1. Readmission rates within 30 days, by diagnosis
2. Readmission rates at 72 hours, by diagnosis
3. Adjusted mortality rates

INPATIENT PHYSICIAN PEOPLE MEASURES:

1. Physician-to-physician peer review. Peer-to-peer review can include:
    a. Primary care physicians review hospitalists
    b. Hospitalists review specialty physicians
    c. Specialty physicians review hospitalists
    d. Hospitalists review ER physicians
    e. ER physicians review hospitalists
    f. Hospitalists review hospitalists
2. Nurse review of physician interaction with nurses
3. Committee participation
4. Meeting attendance

INPATIENT FINANCE MEASURES:

1. Admission history and physicals completed per shift
2. Discharge orders written by noon
3. Length of stay, overall
4. Length of stay by specific diagnosis
5. Total cost per admission
6. Total cost by diagnosis

7. Length of stay outliers (>13 days)

INPATIENT GROWTH MEASURES:

1. Patient likelihood of recommending hospital to others
2. Patient likelihood of recommending physician to others
3. Discharge summaries sent to primary care physicians within 24 hours of discharge

INPATIENT SERVICE MEASURES:

1. How often did your physician treat you with dignity and respect?
2. How often did your physician use language you could easily understand?
3. How often did your physician include you in healthcare decision making?

EMERGENCY ROOM PHYSICIAN PERFORMANCE MEASURES

Physician performance measurement, reporting, and feedback in the emergency room environment can have significant impact on physician behaviors. The encapsulated ER environment with the same group of employed or contracted physicians, like the employed outpatient environment, lends itself well to performance assessment and reporting. Similar methods of goal selection apply to individual physician performance measures in the ER setting, with physician measures "matching" and aligning to system performance goals.

PHYSICIAN EMERGENCY ROOM QUALITY MEASURES:

1. Aspirin on arrival for acute myocardial infarction
2. ECG performed for non-traumatic chest pain
3. ECG performed for syncope patients
4. Vital signs for patients with community-acquired pneumonia (CAP)
5. Oxygen saturations for patients with CAP

6. Assessment of mental status for patients with CAP
7. Appropriate empiric antibiotic for CAP
8. Consider T-PA for ischemic stroke
9. Severe sepsis patients with management order bundle initiated
10. Intubated patients with confirmation of endotracheal tube placement
11. Female patients with abdominal pain have a pregnancy test done
12. Patients with pulmonary embolism have anti-coagulation orders in the ED

PHYSICIAN EMERGENCY ROOM SERVICE MEASURES:

1. How well did the emergency room physician and nurse work together?
2. How well did the ED provider explain your diagnosis?
3. How well did the ED provider manage your pain?
4. How well did your ED provider listen to your concerns?
5. How well did the ED provider explain what was done in the emergency room?
6. Patient complaints per 1,000 ED visits

PHYSICIAN EMERGENCY ROOM PEOPLE MEASURES:

1. ED to ED physician peer review
2. Hospitalist review of ED physicians
3. Specialist review of ED physicians
4. Nurse review of ED physicians

PHYSICIAN EMERGENCY ROOM FINANCE MEASURES:

1. Door to doctor time
2. Patients seen per hour
3. Clinical charges
4. Length of ED stay for discharged patients
5. Patients leaving without being seen
6. Patients leaving against medical advice
7. Discharged patients with ED times exceeding six hours

PHYSICIAN EMERGENCY ROOM GROWTH MEASURES:

1. Likelihood of recommending emergency room to others

CREATING PHYSICIAN SCORECARDS

Measuring physician performance across pillars should be compiled and created as a single-source dashboard of physician performance. These scorecards will serve as the reporting method in which physicians will see their own compiled performance in a single document. It would be a great disservice to the improvement process to select physician performance measures, assess performance across pillars, align measures with organizational goals, and then *fail* to effectively communicate these performance measures to physicians. The influence of performance assessment on physician performance depends on how well results are communicated to physicians.

Several important principles in creating meaningful physician scorecards are:

1. Make scorecards simple and easy to read. Do not give physicians 15-page reports. They are unlikely to read a long, complicated document.
2. Scorecards need to contain physician performance compared to peers and compared to expectations (goals). Both expectations and comparative performance are compelling to physicians and both need to be communicated on a physician scorecard.
3. Report performance over time to identify trends.
4. Communicating physician performance compared to peers can be done several ways:

   a. **Ranking physicians:** Quality and performance measures will generate a list of physicians. This list creates the "rank" of physicians by scores. The individual physician scorecard can present a physician's relative rank within a department.

Ranking is not necessarily transparent, but will show a physician ranked "27th" in a department of 30. This ranking report gives clear, and sometimes brutal, comparative performance, but keeps rankings private.

b. **Physician performance versus system average:** This is a simple way of providing comparative performance measurement across selected pillar goals. Physicians' "self-awareness" of how they compare to peers is the most influential measure in changing physician behavior. High scores yield pride and continued focus on execution. Lower scores, particularly if transparent, yield motivation and effort to make performance better.

ASSEMBLING PHYSICIAN SCORECARDS

Below are examples of compiled physician scorecards that can be used as templates for reporting physician performance across pillars. Scorecards need to be specific for an organization in which reported measures are consistent with organizational goals. Features of these scorecards include:

1. Pillar-based goals
2. Physician performance compared to goals
3. Physician performance compared to peers
4. Performance over time

Figure 6.3

BALANCED OUTPATIENT PHYSICIAN SCORECARD SAMPLE

Pillar	Metric	Peer Avg.	Goal	Jan 08	Mar 08	May 08	Jul 08	Sep 08	YTD
Quality	HgA1c >9	11.2%	**8.0%**	15.8%	16.2%	13.9%	14.6%	13.7%	**14.9%**
	LDL <100 patients with DM	62.0%	**70.0%**	49.0%	48.0%	50.0%	52.0%	54.0%	**51.0%**
	BP <140/90 in HTN	62.0%	**75.0%**	57.0%	60.0%	63.0%	63.0%	68.0%	**62.4%**
	Annual urinary microalbumin screen in patients with DM	72.5%	**85.0%**	69.0%	72.3%	72.9%	74.4%	76.9%	**73.8%**
	Annual influenza vacc in pts > 50	58.0%	**65.0%**	42.0%	48.5%	n/a	n/a	n/a	**48.5%**
	Annual mammogram in women 40-70	71.0%	**90.0%**	55.0%	59.0%	61.0%	63.0%	68.0%	**61.2%**
Service	Patient satisfaction (percentile)	60th percentile	**75th percentile**	17th percentile	20th percentile	24th percentile	24th percentile	31st percentile	**24th percentile**
People	Peer review (1-5)	4.2	**4.5**	3.9	n/a	n/a	n/a	n/a	**4.1**
	Staff review (1-5)	4.0	**4.5**	2.8	n/a	n/a	n/a	n/a	**3.1**
Growth	Likelihood to recommend physician	65th percentile	**75th percentile**	4th percentile	3rd percentile	5th percentile	5th percentile	6th percentile	**5th percentile**
Finance	Patients seen per day	19.0	**22.0**	18.0	19.0	22.0	23.0	23.0	**21.1**

Key

Shade	Meaning
Medium gray	Meeting or exceeding goal
Light gray	Above peer average, below goal
Dark gray	At or below peer average

Figure 6.4

INPATIENT PHYSICIAN SCORECARD SAMPLE

Pillar	Metric	Peer Avg.	Goal	Jan 08	Feb 08	Mar 08	Jul 08	Aug 08	YTD
Quality	ASA at DC for AMI	96.5%	**98.0%**	n/a	91.5%	n/a	n/a	96.0%	**94.2%**
	Beta blocker at DC for AMI	94.0%	**98.0%**	n/a	92.5%	n/a	n/a	94.0%	**93.2%**
	ACE/ARB for LV systolic dysfunction	92.0%	**95.0%**	n/a	88.0%	n/a	n/a	92.4%	**91.8%**
	Appropriate initial antibiotic for CAP	84.0%	**90.0%**	n/a	80.0%	n/a	n/a	84.0%	**82.8%**
	MS exam for CAP	68.0%	**90.0%**	n/a	62.0%	n/a	n/a	68.0%	**67.4%**
Service	Physician listened to patient (% always)	72.0%	**85.0%**	62.0%	66.0%	71.0%	74.0%	70.0%	**69.0%**
	Physician respected patient (% always)	68.0%	**85.0%**	66.0%	70.0%	68.0%	66.0%	68.0%	**70.0%**
	Physician explained so patient understood (% always)	70.0%	**85.0%**	64.0%	62.0%	62.0%	63.0%	69.0%	**68.0%**
People	Peer review (1-5)	4.4	**4.5**	n/a	4.0	n/a	n/a	4.4	**4.3**
	Nurse review (1-5)	4.1	**4.5**	n/a	4.6	n/a	n/a	4.7	**4.8**
	DC summary sent to PCP	78.0%	**90.0%**	n/a	40.0%	44.0%	49.0%	52.5%	**48.2%**
Finance	30-day re-admit rate	12.0%	**8.0%**	n/a	14.0%	12.6%	11.0%	8.0%	**10.2%**
	LOS, overall average	3.61	**3.56**	3.91	3.81	3.69	3.62	3.68	**3.74**
	DC completed by noon	68.0%	**80.0%**	60.0%	68.0%	51.0%	66.0%	69.0%	**68.0%**

Key

(medium shade)	Meeting or exceeding goal
(light shade)	Above peer average, below goal
(dark shade)	At or below peer average

Figure 6.5

ER PHYSICIAN SCORECARD SAMPLE

Pillar	Metric	Peer Avg.	Goal	Jan 08	Feb 08	Mar 08	Apr 08	May 08	Jun 08	Jul 08	Aug 08	Sep 08	YTD
Quality	ASA at arrival for AMI	92.0%	**95.0%**		96.0%			97.0%			96.0%		**96.0%**
	Beta blocker for AMI	93.0%	**95.0%**		92.0%			94.0%			96.0%		**95.0%**
	Blood cultures prior to AB for CAP	90.0%	**95.0%**		78.9%			92.0%			94.0%		**93.0%**
	Antibiotics within 4 hours for CAP	88.0%	**95.0%**		84.0%			88.0%			92.0%		**92.0%**
	EKG for syncope patients	94.0%	**98.0%**		94.0%			94.0%			98.0%		**96.0%**
Service	Patient satisfaction (percentile)	60th percentile	**75th percentile**	68th percentile	78th percentile	80th percentile	82nd percentile	82nd percentile	88th percentile	84th percentile	88th percentile	92nd percentile	**84th percentile**
	Door-to-doc time	46 minutes	**30 minutes**	42 minutes	49 minutes	39 minutes	46 minutes	40 minutes	36 minutes	34 minutes	31 minutes	22 minutes	**36 minutes**
	How well did provider manage pain	60th percentile	**80th percentile**	n/a	72nd percentile	78th percentile	82nd percentile	68th percentile	74th percentile	76th percentile	80th percentile	84th percentile	**82nd percentile**
People	Peer review (1-5)	4.3	**4.5**	n/a	4.1	n/a	n/a	n/a	n/a	n/a	4.2	n/a	**4.2**
	Nurse review (1-5)	4.1	**4.5**	n/a	3.1	n/a	n/a	n/a	n/a	n/a	n/a	n/a	**3.2**
Growth	Left without being seen rate (%)	3.8%	**2.0%**	4.2%	4.0%	3.1%	3.0%	2.2%	2.4%	1.8%	1.6%	2.8%	**3.4%**
Finance	Patients per hour	2.5	**2.7**	2.0	1.3	2.2	2.5	2.6	2.7	2.7	2.8	2.8	**2.4**

Key

Shading	Meaning
Medium gray	Meeting or exceeding goal
Light gray	Above peer average, below goal
Dark gray	At or below peer average

SUMMARY

The extent to which the physician measurement stage is executed as well as an organization's commitment to this process will heavily influence the level of improvement a system is able to achieve. Measurement represents the gears of change, and allows aspiration, motivation, and hope to evolve into a predictable, tactical mechanism to change and align physician behaviors. In the absence of objective performance data, the "argument" and case for change is weak. In the absence of measurement, a physician's self-affirming self-estimate can create assurance that everything is fine, making change and a sense of urgency challenging to achieve. Measurement is the mirror, the foundation, and the reason for doing things differently.

Physicians care deeply about clinical quality, the patient experience, colleague opinion, workplace culture, and how physicians treat and get along with team members. In the intensity of the day, physicians can often lose focus and attention on these critical performance issues. Physicians can become preoccupied with simple perseverance, and gravitate toward old habits and interactions. Measurement and performance feedback, coupled with coaching and training, can lift physicians up, make them better, and keep attention, focus, and effort on the things that matter most.

Key Learnings for Stage 6, "Physician Measurement and Balanced Scorecards":

1. Measurement and reporting of physician performance measures is an important change strategy for physician behaviors.
2. Measurement and reporting of performance provides the "reality" of current performance. Without knowledge of comparative performance, substantive physician change is unlikely.
3. Comparative performance reporting impacts physician behavior more than raw, noncomparative data.
4. Transparent performance measures have more influence on physician behaviors than veiled data.
5. Select goals for physicians across pillars that support and "match" organizational goals.
6. Report physician performance compared to peers and to an expectation (goal).
7. Use a systemic, timely reporting method to physicians in the format of a pillar-based scorecard.

STAGE 7:
Implementing Physician Behavioral Standards

"There can be no happiness if the things we believe in are different from the things that we do."

—Freya Stark

When I wrote *Practicing Excellence: A Physician's Manual to Exceptional Health Care,* I wrote a chapter on creating and implementing behavioral standards for physicians. I chose to include this topic again due to the fact that behavioral standards are going from an elective pursuit deployed by high-performing systems to a Joint Commissions mandate, beginning in 2009. The Joint Commission directive reads:

The Joint Commission is introducing new standards requiring more than 15,000 accredited healthcare organizations to create a code of conduct that defines acceptable and unacceptable behaviors and to establish a formal process for managing unacceptable behavior. The new standards take effect January 1, 2009, for hospitals, nursing homes, home health agencies, laboratories, ambulatory care facilities, and behavioral healthcare facilities across the United States.

Of all the stages of physician engagement that a system implements, rolling out behavioral standards may be the most volatile. Physicians have seen the hospital-created Joint Commissions mandate as a viable threat to their autonomy, with little input into the creation of standards or recourse for "violations" of a code of conduct.

To quote one physician's perspective on the evolving Hospital Code of Conduct, I have included an excerpt from an editorial published in 2008 in the *Journal of Physicians and Surgeons.* Lawrence Huntoon, MD, writes:

"In the never-ending quest of hospital administrations to gain more power and control over physicians on staff, the underlying purpose of imposing a physician code of conduct on physicians is clear—it diminishes the professional standing of physicians on staff and in so doing increases the hospital's authority and control over physicians. The physician code of conduct is intentionally insulting, demeaning, and degrading to physicians, and reduces physicians to being treated like juvenile delinquents at a reform school. It assumes that all physicians, like juvenile delinquents, need to be subjected to a long list of prohibited behaviors because, in the hospital administration's view, physicians are predisposed to such things as theft, destruction of property, and physical and sexual assault."

This oppositional physician perception and opinion is not uncommon. Not infrequently, codes of conduct are seen by physicians as simply being unilateral mechanisms intended to rid a system of physician whistleblowers.

The intent, goals, and spirit of physician behavioral standards are clearly not designed to create suspicion and distrust between medical staff and system administration. Unfortunately, if this stage is not done properly, it has the potential to poison physician relations and to create a chasm between physicians and administrative leaders.

The diagnostic evaluation of systems in which physicians attack the prospect of behavioral standards is most often a testimony to the history and pre-existing relationship between the medical staff and the administration. If a chilled relationship is in place, then hospital-driven behavioral standards will be met with rejection and distrust. The prospect of proceeding with behavioral standards without a foundation of strong physician relations will be fraught with headache. The centerpiece of effective physician engagement is a trusting, responsive, efficient, collaborative environment in which vision and culture are clear and where performance, accountability, and execution are embedded at every level of the system. If Stages 1 through 6 are implemented, behavioral standards will be seen as a logical progression in the evolution, maturation, and growth of the system.

Behavioral standards for physicians are sequenced late in the physician engagement process by design. Behavioral standards should be implemented when the appropriate organizational "pre-work" has been completed. The following conditions should be in place prior to launching a physician code of conduct:

1. Organizational vision is clear, communicated to, and supported by the medical staff.
2. System pillar goals are in place and are understood.

3. A "you spoke, we responded" experience is in place for members of the medical staff.
4. Leaders round on physicians to build relationships, establish communication, and respond to practice concerns.
5. Physician leaders are firmly aligned to organizational vision and goals.
6. Consensus is established between physician and administrative leaders regarding vision, goals, and strategies.
7. Physician champions are selected, developed, and deployed.
8. A code of conduct is in place for the administrative team. Nothing will foster physician suspicion more than the perception that physicians are being singled out. There are many systems that will use an organizationwide code of conduct that is applied to every member of the healthcare team.
9. Physicians are trained by physician champions in behaviors consistent with the new code of conduct.

Even after building a strong foundation toward physician engagement, skill and finesse are still necessary in effectively rolling out and implementing these standards of conduct. The following is a sequenced pathway designed to optimize effectiveness, support, and impact while minimizing physician protest.

PHYSICIAN BEHAVIORAL STANDARDS ROLLOUT SEQUENCE

1. Assemble physician leaders and respected informal physician leaders to draft behavioral standards.
   a. Physician suspicion of standards is diminished and physician leader "ownership" is enhanced when physicians create the standards.
   b. Select physicians who have the respect of the medical staff and who are aligned with the system vision to draft standards. These assembled physicians will not only be

tasked with creating standards, but should be the voice used in communicating standards to the general medical staff.

2. Determine a profile of desired and unacceptable behaviors. It is suggested that physicians respond more positively to what we "aspire to do" versus "what you cannot do."

3. Physician members of the behavioral standards committee must learn and appreciate that it is *what they say* and *how they communicate* this code of conduct to their colleagues that will determine the physician response. Even well-written codes of conduct can have little impact on physician behavior. The impact of behavioral standards on physician behaviors is significantly influenced by how the code of conduct is positioned and presented. The physician leaders' communication of behavioral standards should include the following:
   a. No apologies. If a physician leader is tentative and reserved in regards to the standards content, the standards will be disregarded and ignored by the medical staff.
   b. Communicate standards as "who we are." If all prior stages of physician engagement have been completed, physicians should expect, understand, and even endorse this physician-created code of conduct.
   c. Communication of behavioral standards should come in comprehensive "multi-channel" formats. (See Stage 1 to review multi-channel communication.) Leaders must understand that a system has behavioral standards only if physicians have seen them and know what they are, and if they impact what physicians do. Use the following strategies to communicate behavioral standards to the medical staff:

i. Medical staff meetings
ii. Physician newsletters
iii. Rounding on physicians
iv. Physician orientation
v. Physician training

After the communication and rollout of behavioral standards, there is value and impact in projecting a code of conduct where patients will see it. Banner Health, Desert Samaritan Medical Center Emergency Department utilized this principle when it created a "Performance Guarantee" for Clinical Excellence and Exceptional Customer Service with specific behavioral commitments to its emergency room patients. This code of conduct was framed, illuminated, signed by every care provider (including physicians), and placed prominently in the patient reception area. A code of conduct is more likely to influence physicians if standards are expressed as a visible and genuine commitment to patients, signed by physicians, and profiled at the center of the care environment.

The code of conduct is the communication of expectations that are intended to create behavioral consistency within the medical staff. The code of conduct distills the system vision and physician training to simple behaviors reflective of the physician role in organizational change. The code of conduct aims high and makes clear what should and cannot occur. Behavioral standards cultivate physician conduct that builds enduring patient loyalty, marketplace differentiation, workplace partnership, and a culture of safety and performance.

In order for a system to change culture and develop a "brand" of extraordinary care, the system must do what it says it will do all the time. To do something all the time, it must be clear *what* it is that will be done all of the time. Consistency of behavior must become so embedded that patients begin to "expect" and anticipate being taken care of in a certain way, regardless of which department, nurse, or individual physician they see. Great systems differentiate themselves from others not just by doing things better, but by doing things every time. Organizational reputations are built through predictability and consistency. A visible, palpable, trained, and embraced code of conduct must be in place to create consistency and predictability and to execute the "always" culture.

CONTENT OF PHYSICIAN BEHAVIORAL STANDARDS

As an organization begins to write or rewrite a code of conduct, it must decide which behaviors to place in this document. The final content of the behavioral standards will ultimately rest with those drafting the document. The Joint Commissions have issued a Sentinel Event Alert identifying disruptive and rude behaviors as a direct threat to safety and quality and have provided a framework of content, which standards of conduct need to address. Guidelines provided by Joint Commissions to assist in the implementation of behavioral standards include the following:

Recommendations from Joint Commissions' Code of Conduct:

1. Educate all healthcare team members about professional behavior, including training in basics such as being courteous during telephone interactions, business etiquette, and general people skills.
2. Hold all team members accountable for modeling desirable behaviors and enforce the code of conduct consistently and equitably.
3. Establish a comprehensive approach to addressing intimidating and disruptive behaviors. This approach should include a zero-tolerance policy that relies on strong involvement and support from physician leadership.
4. Create policy that reduces the fear of retribution against those who report intimidating and disruptive behaviors.

5. Empathize with and apologize to patients and families who are involved in or witness intimidating or disruptive behaviors.
6. Determine how and when disciplinary actions should begin.
7. Develop a system to detect and receive reports of unprofessional behavior. Use non-confrontational interaction strategies to address intimidating and disruptive behaviors within the context of an organizational commitment to the health and well-being of all staff and patients.

Examples of "unacceptable" and "desired" behaviors that can be included in a physician code of conduct are referenced below:

Unacceptable Physician Behaviors:

- Shouting or yelling
- Use of profanity directed at another individual or healthcare professional
- Slamming or throwing objects in anger or disgust
- Hostile, condemning, or demeaning communications
- Criticism of performance and/or competency delivered in an inappropriate location (i.e., not in private) and not aimed at performance improvement
- Other behavior demonstrating disrespect, intimidation, or disruption to the delivery of quality patient care
- Retaliation against any person who addresses or reports unacceptable behavior
- Criticizing the care provided by a physician colleague in the written medical record or in a public place

Expected Physician Behaviors:

Interaction with staff

- Recognize that every member of the team is important and makes an important contribution to patient care.

- Be available and cooperative when on call. When paged, respond promptly and appropriately.
- Communications, including spoken remarks, written documents, and e-mails, should be honest and direct and should be conducted in a professional, constructive, respectful, and efficient manner.
- Provide constructive feedback in the spirit of improvement and in private if inappropriate staff behaviors are observed.

Interaction with physician colleagues

- Make time for direct doctor-to-doctor communication for emergent/urgent consultations.
- Respond affably and as promptly as possible to requests for assistance from a colleague.
- Work in a collegial manner with physician colleagues.
- Treat referring providers with an appropriate spirit of accommodation and service.
- Position physician colleagues positively to patients as a referring or consultant physician.
- Reference the care and work-up done by other physicians who are providing care to a patient to improve the sense of continuity.

Interaction with patients

- Knock on the door prior to entering an exam room.
- Introduce yourself to patients and family members and explain your role in the care team.
- Wear your ID badge above the waist so that patients and others can see it.
- Smile, make eye contact, and address patients by name. Realize that body language and tone of voice are important parts of communication.
- Thank patients for waiting if you are running late.

- Wash your hands before and after every patient contact to reduce the spread of infection.
- Respect patient privacy: use curtains and doors, ask permission prior to removing garments, and conduct conversations in private areas.
- Learn about the patient as a person, not just as a diagnosis.
- Each patient is an individual and should be treated with respect and kindness.
- Explain treatment needs, treatment options, and potential treatment outcomes in a way that the patient can understand.
- Explain medications so that patients will understand the purpose of the medication, how long they will take it, and what the potential side effects might be.
- Explain a patient's diagnosis using simple language he or she will understand.
- Include the patient opinion and preference for health outcomes when determining the best treatment plan.

USING A CODE OF CONDUCT TO CHANGE PHYSICIAN BEHAVIOR

It is fairly clear that many codes of conduct are written and subsequently have little impact on physician behavior. A true code of conduct exists only if it changes what physicians do. How the code of conduct is communicated and positioned by physician and executive leadership is as important as the content of behavioral standards. Here are guidelines to using the physician-created code of conduct to align physician behavior to the system culture:

1. Physician leadership must communicate the content of behavioral standards to the medical staff. Administrative leadership doing this without physicians at the lead is likely to meet resistance.

2. Make the case for physician behavior not as a pawn in a hospital agenda, but as a necessity for patient safety, clinical quality, and physician practice success.
3. If inherent resistance is sensed, use compelling, real examples of specific physician behaviors that clearly violate system standards and that illustrate the impact of physician conduct on patients, staff, families, and the organization.
4. Use the code of conduct as a tool in the interview process when selecting employed physicians. The desired behaviors in the code of conduct become the selection criteria and behavioral "profile" for new physicians joining the system.
5. Physician orientation, both with new employed or affiliated physicians, should have specific, clear exposure to the code of conduct. The code of conduct has the greatest influence during the initiation and orientation of physicians into the organization and its culture.
6. Be very clear: The code of conduct is how the organization is run, and collaborative and respectful physician behavior is a requisite for a clinical work environment that is marked by safety, quality, and service. Violations of the code of conduct must have consequences. (See Stage 8, "Managing the Disruptive Physician.") If a code of conduct has no teeth, it is not a code of conduct.
7. Have physicians sign the code of conduct to improve awareness and knowledge of its content and to raise accountability for compliance. Signing can be done while applying for privileges or during recredentialing.
8. Use the code of conduct for physician training. Training and development will be ongoing (see Stage 5, "Training Physicians"), and using your behavioral standards as a template for training content will keep physicians aware of conduct standards.

9. Place the code of conduct in a place where patients can see it, preferably signed by all of the medical staff leadership. Use behavioral standards to make a strong and visible gesture that conveys "who we are." When specific behaviors are highly visible, are placed on the wall, and are signed by physicians, consistency and accountability for adherence is raised.

As behavioral standards are rolled out to the medical staff, one of the most important and predictive conditions of receptiveness is what physicians see system leaders do. If leader conduct is not aligned with stated standards for physicians, physicians will categorically reject those standards. Leaders cannot ask anyone else to comply with system behaviors if they do not engage in those behaviors themselves.

Key Learnings for Stage 7, "Implementing Physician Behavioral Standards":

1. A code of conduct and a policy for response to a violation of a code of conduct will be organizational requirements for those systems regulated by Joint Commissions in 2009.
2. A code of conduct represents specific physician behaviors that are consistent with the vision and mission of the organization. The articulated code of conduct represents clear communication of the physician role in an organizational change effort.
3. The code of conduct should be written and communicated by respected physician leaders and colleagues.
4. Physician leaders who create the code of conduct will select unacceptable and expected physician behaviors when establishing the content of behavioral standards.
5. A code of conduct has greater impact on physician behaviors when it is:
   a. Created by physicians.
   b. Presented by physician leaders as important with a firm commitment to "who we are."
   c. Used for physician orientation.
   d. Signed by physicians during privileging or recredentialing.
   e. Included as part of physician training (see Stage 5, "Training Physicians").
   f. Not just a set of guidelines. Consequences should be in place for violations of the code of conduct (see Stage 8, "Managing the Disruptive Physician").
   g. Placed in a high-visibility area where patients, staff, and physicians can clearly see the code of conduct.

STAGE 8:
Managing the Disruptive Physician

"There is only do and do not—there is no try."

—Yoda

The management of disruptive physicians can be one of the most challenging responsibilities for medical staff leadership. Most physician leaders perceive disruptive behavior intervention to be intrinsically oppositional, and it usually ranks at the top of the list of most dreaded leader activities. The pathway to managing difficult physicians must be proactive, consistent, and deliberate, and should be activated when the clearly communicated, signed physician behavior standards are violated.

DEFINITION

The definition of disruptive behavior is often non-specific and vague. Clarity of disruptive behaviors is substantially improved with articulated system behavioral standards that clearly communicate what should and cannot happen. The American Medical Association (AMA) has defined disruptive behavior as "a style of interaction with physicians, hospital personnel, patients, family members, or others that interferes with patient care." The profile of physician disruptive behaviors is broad and far more subtle than the hurling of instruments. The spectrum of disruptive behaviors may include the following:

- Unwillingness to adhere to practice policies
- Failure to respond to pages that compromises care delivery to patients
- Constant tardiness
- Disorganized and unable to maintain a schedule
- Unprofessional appearance or demeanor
- Poor bedside manner
- Unwillingness to see a full patient load, help out in a pinch, or assume responsibility
- Clinical "laziness"—not interested in keeping up on advances in the field
- Stubborn and inflexible
- Argumentative (always right, never wrong)
- Complaining to patients, staff, or other physicians outside the group about colleagues and internal matters
- Using critical, derogatory, foul, or crude language
- Inappropriate expressions of anger, resentment, extreme negativity, moodiness, or irritability
- Threats of violence or legal action directed at staff, partners, or patients
- Offensive humor, sexual innuendo, or sexual harassment
- Belittling or intimidating fellow healthcare team members, including physician colleagues, ancillary, or nursing staff

The spirit of managing disruptive physicians is simply to uphold conduct consistent with the vision and culture of the institution. Managing disruptive physicians is not designed nor intended to muzzle opinion, stifle out of the box thinking, or blunt expression of thoughts. Behavioral intervention is not meant to attack a physician who works with an intensity many will never know or who may be crumbling under personal duress and taking it out on those around him.

When violations of a code of conduct occur, action and communication from leadership must follow. Reaching out and helping struggling physicians is worth every ounce of organizational resources used, and should be the driving principle behind a disruptive physician strategy. Though help and assistance to struggling physicians spearhead the effort, behaviors to support safety, respect, collaboration, and team are not optional or "negotiable." The character and culture of the organization are at stake. Others are watching, and an acceptance and tolerance of toxic physician behaviors will strike at the credibility and fortitude of leaders and call into question the commitment and backbone of the leadership team. No one wins when physicians are lost, but losing physicians is sometimes necessary.

IMPACT OF THE DISRUPTIVE PHYSICIAN

The impact of unmanaged disruptive behaviors can be devastating. Systems can invest in new facilities, staff training, recruitment, and expanding service lines, but all efforts can be undone by failing to control physicians' mean-spirited, destructive behaviors. In the age of the Internet and the prospect of rapid, unlimited information dissemination, patients and staff can threaten an entire institution by testimonies of unmanaged, disruptive physicians. The culture of the system will ultimately be defined by the conduct of its physicians, and the strength of leadership will be judged by the ability to act fairly, consistently, and decisively when disruptive physician behaviors arise.

The leader struggle with difficult physicians is waged in healthcare systems across the country. In a survey of 1,627 physician executives, 96 percent reported regularly encountering disruptive physician behavior, and 70 percent said disruptive behaviors nearly always involved the same physicians. Common disruptive behaviors were disrespect, refusal to complete tasks and carry out duties, yelling, insults, and physical abuse (including throwing items). A majority (57 percent) reported that disruptive physician behaviors most often involved conflict with a nurse or other allied healthcare staff. Other respondents said disruptive behaviors most often involved other physicians (15 percent), administrators (14 percent), and patients (14 percent). Notably, nearly 80 percent of the respondents said that disruptive physician behavior is under-reported because of victim fear of reprisal, or is reported only when a serious violation occurs.[25]

In a 2004 survey of over 1,500 nurses and 350 pharmacists, the Institute for Safe Medication Practices reported that nearly half of nurses and pharmacists admitted that physician intimidation had changed how they handled questions about medication orders. Forty percent reported having concerns about the safety of a medication at least once in the past year and assumed it was correct rather than interacting with an intimidating prescriber.

Disruptive physicians undermine morale, diminish productivity and the quality of patient care, and cause work environment distress leading to heightened employee turnover.[26, 27] One survey found that most nurses believe physician disruptive behavior causes stress, frustration, impaired concentration, reduced collaboration and communication, and negative patient outcomes. Another survey found that nurses see a direct link between physician disruptive behavior and nurse satisfaction, retention, and the quality of the nurse-physician relationship.[28, 29]

Although quality and work environment are the most visible and frequently cited casualties of disruptive physician behavior, the potential impact can ripple further. Attending physicians who exhibit abusive behavior to residents tend to create residents who display similar behaviors.[30] Leader physicians with abusive styles will breed physician isolation and withdrawal in which physicians begin to lose the spirit of caring for others and exhibit a diminished willingness to participate in system activities. Physicians subject to abusive colleagues will withdraw from the toxic environment and become concerned only with protecting themselves. As physicians have grown increasingly dependent on each other for expertise, referrals, procedures, committees, and initiatives, progress will be difficult if these disruptive conditions and individuals are left unbridled. Building a culture of excellence demands building a culture of communication, character, respect, collaboration, and a willingness to work together.

Disruptive physicians who protest efforts, criticize colleagues, and disrespect patients will distract and stall system efforts. If left unaddressed, difficult physician behavior will create a firm platform on which other non-physician staff can stand and enact the same. Nothing validates, legitimizes, and accelerates complaining and protest more than the example set by the unmanaged disruptive physician. Counteracting the potential direct and indirect impacts of disruptive behavior requires understanding, proactive action, and consistently applied strategy to preserve system culture from the influence of a vocal few.

THE PROFILE OF THE DISPRUPTIVE PHYSICIAN

It is estimated that 80 percent of physicians never have an incidence of disruptive behavior at any time during their careers. Another 16 to 18 percent will have a singular event, provoked by circumstances or personal issues. Two to four percent of physicians will display disruptive behavior as a repeated behavioral pattern.[31] The nature of disruptive physician intervention will be based on the stratification of whether or not a physician's behaviors represent an aberrancy or a repeated behavioral cycle.

Those physicians who exhibit repeated patterns of disruptive behavior typically show little insight into their own behaviors, deflecting responsibility to everyone but themselves. They tend to hold high self-opinions, sometimes bordering on narcissistic, and view the world around them as categorically incompetent. They tend to think that they are the smartest physicians around, and sometimes they are. Clinical talent is a common feature of disruptive physicians. They tend to have short fuses, requiring very little provocation to set them off. They have poor abilities to manage and control anger. Disruptive physicians are typically lonely, frequently having burned colleague and administrative support networks that would otherwise come to the aid of a struggling physician. These physicians will often find a susceptible colleague to "confide" in, and will self-create allegiances in which to vent and voice their disdain for others.

A disruptive physician rarely "flips a switch" and becomes disruptive when he or she joins a medical staff. The disruptive physician likely has behavior patterns that date back to medical school or earlier. Those in charge of physician appointments and credentialing should be trained and developed to query and identify physicians' past behaviors. A physician's prior behavior will predict his or her future conduct. Frequently (and unfortunately) these physicians have been unchallenged, or have rolled over trivial efforts to correct their destructive behaviors.

Intervention for disruptive physicians must be in place and must be consistent. The prospect of disruptive physician intervention may keep leaders awake at night, but this can pale in comparison to the prospective impact of inactivity. This is not an easy undertaking, but apprehension of this critical effort is not a justification for failing to respond, and it is the responsibility of the leadership team to move. A consistent disruptive physician leader response system must be put into place to enforce a code of conduct. The potential consequences of silence can jeopardize the entire enterprise—the voice and strength of leadership are required.

DISRUPTIVE PHYSICIAN INTERVENTION

In years past, the overarching approach to disruptive physician behavior has been, "He's a jerk, and we need to get rid of him." Although these actions are sometimes necessary, stripping a physician of his or her livelihood should not be the aim or intention of leaders committed to managing difficult physicians. A newer and refreshed paradigm is to help physicians re-establish a successful clinical practice and restore their professional standing as productive members of the medical staff. Nobody wins when a physician's privileges are lost. The loss of a physician can be devastating to the physician and costly to the organization. Intervention for disruptive physicians is intended to maintain physician clinical activity without compromising safety, quality, and the work environment that is at the foundation of system efforts and culture. If the intervention of disruptive physicians results in the loss of a physician, the system and approach has failed in its intention.

Every stage articulated in this manual is intended to prevent and preempt disruptive physician behavior before it manifests. These efforts include:

- Communicating a clear vision that is boldly projected throughout the system, which is dedicated to patients, employees, and physicians and establishes the aspirations and expectations of the system.
- Creating a high-performance clinical environment dedicated to physician efficiency, superior outcomes, and system responsiveness to physicians' concerns that builds physician trust and confidence in the leadership team.
- Creating a system in which the physician voice is heard, effective leaders are in place, and physician champions are activated. This establishes a sense of physician involvement and partnership.

- Training and investing in the improvement of physicians as a sincere, collaborative gesture to physicians in order to promote their success.
- A clearly articulated, physician-developed code of conduct consistent with the vision and culture of the system.

These progressive stages of physician engagement have the power to cool animosity, heal wounds, demonstrate performance, foster collaboration, establish accountability, and develop a culture in which disruptive behavior is far less likely to emerge.

Despite efforts to prevent disruptive behavior, it is still going to happen. A deliberate, consistent policy to deal with it must be in place. The following steps represent an outline of intervening when a violation of a communicated code of conduct arises.

IDENTIFY THE DISRUPTIVE EVENT

The principal purpose of a code of conduct is to convey expectations. The presence of a well-communicated and understood code of conduct serves not only as a disruptive behavior prevention strategy, but also improves the ability to identify disruptive behaviors when they occur. When expectations are effectively conveyed, clearly articulated, and signed by physicians, there is less ambiguity regarding behaviors that should and should not happen.

Communicating expectations to physicians is a key element that proactively reduces disruptive behaviors and develops a culture of safety, respect, and effective communication among healthcare team members. As standards are rolled out, it is essential to develop concurrent strategies and policies that provide clear directive to properly look into reports of disruptive behaviors and clear violations of a code of conduct. All team members, each of whom is held to similar standards, must feel safe and supported by leadership should violations of the code of conduct be reported. This safety provision is a key element of and requirement for effective standards. Reports of disruptive behaviors must be looked into and feedback provided to those individuals reporting behaviors.

A violation of a system code of conduct must have a response. Violations cannot be ignored or brushed off, regardless of who the offender may be. Leader action and intervention needs to be based on a clear breach of behavioral standards, and not just reserved for egregious violations. The nature and type of leader intervention will be influenced by a physician's history of behavior and whether an event is a repeated pattern of conduct or a singular aberrant event. With either scenario, a leader's response must be consistent and predictable. A leader does no one any favors by letting behaviors slide because of the inherent discomfort in having difficult conversations. Behaviors that are not addressed are more likely to continue.

STRATIFY THE DISRUPTIVE EVENT

Categorize disruptive behavior as "singular" or "recurrent." These are different leader conversations with different action plans.

Singular Events: These events tend to happen with physicians who usually do not exhibit disruptive behaviors, but can "crack" under personal or environmental stressors. Nonetheless, these events require leaders to approach and review behaviors with the physician. This intervention is relatively unstructured, and is not in any way meant to be disciplinary or punitive. The phrase "cup of coffee" has been coined by the Joint Commissions to symbolize the casual tenor of this conversation. The "cup of coffee" approach comes from the original work of Vanderbilt's Gerald Hickson, MD, a pioneer in the field of disruptive colleagues and malpractice risk assessment.

Profile of a singular occurrence disruptive physician intervention:

1. **Who:** The intervention for a disruptive physician is done by a physician leader.

2. **What:** The intention of the physician leader approach is to create physician awareness that a specific behavior fell outside of a communicated, understood, and trained code of conduct.

3. **How:** The physician leader approaches the physician and will set the stage. "Joe, there is something important I need to speak with you about. Is now a good time?" You will have the physician's attention at this point. "Yesterday, our charge nurse noted that you had really given a hard time to our travel nurse while you were on call. More specifically, she noted that you were yelling at her and others because you couldn't find a chart, and then yelled at her again when you found out that the patient had gone down to CT before you had a chance to round. Joe, you have been an outstanding member of our medical staff for many years and this is not like you. Is everything okay?"

   Frequently, this dialogue provokes remorse from physicians who respond to the realization of what occurred. "I want to get your side." This query of the physician perspective offers some additional insight into circumstances and can provide a legitimate opportunity for physician input and system improvement. "Is there anything that we can do to prevent this from happening again?" This discussion affirms that the event was noted, and is serious enough to be having this conversation.

   Conclude the conversation with a restatement of the depth of the organizational commitment to a culture of safety and respect with all team members. It is best to finish by articulating a shared goal to align physicians and system intentions. "Joe, you have been on staff here for years and I know that you are committed to a workplace where nurses do not fear physicians. When nurses are intimidated by physicians, the flow of information and patient care is compromised, and I know that we both want the best care for patients."

4. **Result:** Many disruptive physicians will become reflective when physician leaders create awareness of their disruptive behavior and its potential impact on the organization. A simple, honest, and sincere interaction for a first occurrence will often decrease the likelihood of the incident progressing to recurrent disruptive behaviors.

An outline of singular intervention is included:

1. Approach the physician and ask, "Is this a good time?" This approach is equivalent to "permission to speak freely."
2. Articulate specific observed behaviors.
3. Communicate potential impact on the organization.
4. Affirm the physician and recognize contributions that he or she has made to the organization.
5. Get the physician's "side."
6. Articulate the commitment to the organizational code of conduct and reaffirm organizational expectations.
7. Create a shared goal that aligns the physician and organization.

Recurrent Disruptive Behaviors: Recurrent disruptive physician behaviors are more challenging, and likely predate the preventative strategies deployed in prior stages of this manual. It will be no mystery as to who these offenders are, and intervention must occur within close proximity to a recurrent disruptive event. Strike when the iron is warm and not hot. Allow time for emotion and anger to taper prior to approaching disruptive physicians.

1. **Who:** Again, physician leaders will spearhead this intervention. This conversation should not be done alone and should include leaders of departments that are directly involved in the disruptive behavior event. If the event was a physician/nurse interaction, then the chief nursing officer should be involved. A physician leader will need backup and witnesses to make a strong case for this intervention. Witnesses with excellent testimony and specific documentation of events can reduce the risk of a "he said, she said" exchange.

2. **What:** The intention of this interaction is to make clear what happened. The conversation is one of reporting facts and not of passing judgment. The reporting of facts should make clear the impact of the cited behaviors. Disruptive physicians need to understand that their behaviors are not occurring in a bubble, but are rippling throughout the organization with far-reaching effects. Make the impact compelling and sugarcoat nothing. You need to hit disruptive physicians hard enough to generate insight and reflection into their stubborn dispositions.

3. **How:** Make an appointment that will include the physician and the proper support personnel to accompany the physician leader. Do not make small talk. Get right to the point. "Bob, the purpose of this meeting is to address your conduct in the operating room three days ago. It was witnessed that you were screaming at the OR tech because the room had a slow turnaround and made you late for a personal appointment. We also have witnesses who report that you were similarly screaming at another nurse for repeating all medication orders to you over the phone, which is exactly what she is supposed to do. Your behavior is a risk for patient safety and will damage the reputation of this organization for our current workforce and for prospective nurses in this very tight nursing market." Leaders

should cite as many examples as are needed in order to make an overwhelming case for doing things differently. The optimal outcome for these conversations is that the physician reflects and takes responsibility for what he or she has done.

If this is a long-standing pattern of behaviors that has not historically been dealt with, do not expect insight and responsibility to come even from the most compelling of cases. The tenor and action of the conversation must state that no one is exempt from behaving in a way that protects the safety of patients.

This discussion between the physician leader, support personnel, and the disruptive physician is a formal intervention and should be done in accordance with up-to-date bylaws. Inform this physician that repeated patterns of conduct will result in disciplinary action that can include restriction or loss of privileges. Though this conversation is difficult, it is done to create honest and frank communication regarding the seriousness of the cited conduct.

4. **Helping Disruptive Physicians:** The intention of physician intervention is to help, train, and realign physicians so they can continue to practice medicine as members of the medical staff. Resources must be deployed to help, but they need to be administered on the institution's terms. If repeated behaviors that fail to respond to awareness discussions are noted, third-party physician evaluation and training can be accessed. A variety of excellent programs are available, including the PACE program at the University of California in San Diego, California, Vanderbilt Comprehensive Assessment Program for Professionals in Nashville, Tennessee (www.mc.vanderbilt.edu/root/vcap), Pine Grove Professional Enhancement Program in Hattiesburg, Mississippi, and the

Professional Renewal Center in Lawrence, Kansas (www.prckansas.org).

The likelihood of physician change and response to coaching and treatment is directly related to physicians' insight into their own behaviors and the extent to which they assume responsibility for their actions. If they go to training in absolute denial that their actions got them into this situation, the prognosis for significant, sustainable behavioral change is low.

5. **Result:** The goal of intervention for physicians with repeated patterns of disruptive behavior is to provide clear communication of specific physician conduct and its prospective and compelling impact on patients, staff, and the organization. The intervention must include a zero-tolerance message for ongoing behaviors and clear expectations for members of the medical staff consistent with a code of conduct. Resources should be accessed to help physicians, with the expectation and intention of resolving disruptive conduct. If physicians refuse assistance and help, that may be grounds for revoking hospital privileges.

DISRUPTIVE PHYSICIAN HELP

The spirit of the disruptive physician response is to firmly uphold the code of conduct and to do everything possible to minimize conditions that can stir hostile physician behavior. The intent is to offer help and provide resources for physicians so that they become insightful toward their own conduct in order to preserve physician clinical activity. Conversely, physician and administrative leaders must be willing to make hard decisions even for high-revenue-producing physicians.

After the conversation with those with recurrent behavior issues, third-party efforts should be directed at screening and evaluation for treatable causes for behavioral patterns. These include depression, anxiety, personal stressors, medication addiction, alcohol abuse, and medical conditions. Nothing is more tragic than overlooking an easily treatable condition, only to punish the victim by taking away his or her livelihood. For those physicians who want help, no resource should be spared to restore and integrate them back into a successful practice.

Not long ago, an emergency room physician was reported to the Medical Executive Committee of his hospital for being excessively rude and derogatory toward intoxicated patients in his emergency department. The charge nurse in the ER spoke with him about his behavior, but his pattern of conduct continued. This ER physician eventually had his privileges temporarily suspended and was sent for a third-party assessment. During this evaluation process, routine screening assessments were done to assess circumstances and conditions that may have precipitated and contributed to recurrent, disruptive behaviors. During this evaluation it was discovered that the physician's wife had been seriously injured by a drunk driver the previous year. This physician had unknowingly and unintentionally brought this to work with him every day. He was assessed, treated, and has now returned to his successful emergency room practice.

The organizational culture of help and assistance for disruptive physicians should be a simple extension of all that physicians have seen and experienced in the sequenced stages of physician engagement. The culture of an institution that seeks to collaborate with physicians must be firm in its commitment to its vision and character such that physicians hear the following message from physician and executive leadership:

"Our commitment to you is that nobody at the medical center has a title so senior or is a doctor who brings in so much money that he or she is exempt from behaving properly."

The communication and consistency of intervention for disruptive physician behavior is, in and of itself, a preventative strategy. Physicians' awareness of leadership's intense commitment to a culture of safe conduct and the visibility of leader response will create pause for most physicians with behavioral dispositions. If physician behaviors continue to "break through," third-party referral may be necessary, depending on the nature of the offense. Categories of problematic physician conduct and behaviors can include the following:

1. **Anger Management:** Inappropriate expression of anger creates increased staff turnover, low morale, decreased information flow, and patient safety concerns. Physician assistance can help to control physician outbursts.

2. **Physician/Patient Communication:** Poor "bedside manner" diminishes patient satisfaction, patient loyalty, market share, revenue, and system reputation. Poor communication with patients also compromises adherence to medical regimens and raises malpractice risk. Intervention for physicians who struggle with patient interactions can be done on a third-party basis, or by an internal physician champion trained to coach physicians.

3. **Medical Record Keeping:** When physicians have and keep deficient records, the physician and the system are placed at risk for litigation. Third-party physician training can improve record

keeping by providing guidance and standards for adequate documentation.

4. **Inappropriate Prescribing:** Patterns of controlled drug use that are out of compliance with guidelines in prescribing controlled drugs is a physician behavior pattern that can raise concerns at the state board licensing level and can impact care to patients. Physician training can assist physicians with appropriate prescribing patterns and documentation based on care guidelines.

5. **Violation of Professional Boundaries:** Sexual harassment and misconduct and the violation of physician professional boundaries are issues that can place the entire enterprise at risk when physicians are not sufficiently managed by leadership. Physicians who participate in these behaviors will need third-party evaluation and treatment.

PHYSICIAN RE-ENTRY

When physicians successfully undergo third-party intervention, the probability of recurrence of disruptive behaviors declines, and physicians can return to the system. The re-entry process must be structured and clearly communicated to ensure that the same events are not repeated. Re-entry is a conditional process on the institution's terms. The re-entry requirements must be consistent with systemwide behavioral standards. These signed behavioral contracts must be in place with provisions stating that recurrent episodes will not occur. All documented processes must be in accordance with current bylaws of the system.

SUMMARY

The system response to disruptive physician behavior will test the depth and mettle of an organizational commitment more so than any other component of system change. Failure to consistently execute on this front will diminish leaders' ability to create meaningful cultural change elsewhere. Every member of the healthcare team must display vigor of commitment as well as a willingness to do whatever it takes to embed excellence and deliver accountability for everyone. Everyone is worthy of help, but no one is completely untouchable.

Key Learnings for Stage 8, "Managing the Disruptive Physician":

1. Managing disruptive behaviors is based on leader action that upholds a code of conduct.
2. Action for disruptive behaviors needs to be consistent and proactive when a code of conduct is violated.
3. The design and intent of a disruptive physician policy should place its greatest effort and resources toward prevention by executing all stages of physician engagement.
4. Do not wait for egregious violations of behavioral standards before leadership intervention occurs.
5. Perceived inconsistency or tolerance of repeated violations of a code of conduct will make administration of standards much more challenging for leadership. Credibility will be lost.
6. Silence is consent. If a violation occurs and nothing is done, a system does not have a code of conduct.
7. Most physicians will respond to an "awareness" intervention done proactively by a respected physician colleague to create awareness of behaviors and their potential impact on patients, staff, and the organization.
8. If repeated violations continue, intervention is mandatory and is frequently done on a third-party basis.
9. Intervention for help is dependent on the type of violations and should be done on the institution's terms.
10. Intervention is not a formal precursor to physician termination, but is a sincere investment in physician improvement.
11. If physicians fail to respond to third-party assistance or refuse to accept any responsibility for cited conduct, be prepared and willing to lose those physicians.

STAGE 9: RECOGNIZING PHYSICIANS

"Silent gratitude isn't much use to anyone."

—G.B. Stern

I recently did a leadership retreat for a very high-performing healthcare system with top quartile clinical quality indicators, top 10 percent patient satisfaction, and improving physician satisfaction. Certain select, non-leadership physicians were invited to attend this retreat to see the direction, vision, and strategy of the organization as it moved forward. We reviewed the importance of building physician confidence, trust, and partnership to improve the system's ability to initiate quality, safety, and service efforts. During this presentation, a surgeon in the back of the room raised his hand and stood. He told the room how important the efforts of the organization were and how he wanted this sort of service and quality for his patients. He then said that he found it odd that in his five years on the medical staff, despite the millions of dollars of revenue he brought to the institution, no one from the leadership team had ever called him, contacted him, thanked him, or regarded him in any way. He explained how much more willing he would be to truly participate in system efforts if he felt that the "intentions" and words of the leadership team were actually supported by actions.

The recognition of physicians is more important than many leaders realize, and is a frequently overlooked strategy to engage physicians and earn their loyalty. Making a deliberate effort to recognize physicians can and will change the physician perception of a system and its leaders. How do physicians feel about a leader who pulls them aside to thank them for what they do and profiles their recognition to others? Leaders who make a physician look good and feel appreciated will create a physician who is more supportive of the leader's efforts.

Recognition also serves as a physician behavioral change strategy. When physicians are thanked and profiled for doing something, that something is more likely to be repeated. Ninety-three percent of recognized workplace behaviors are replicated,[32] yet many leaders will repeatedly overlook and fail to recognize the very behaviors that created the system's success.

At a recent Sharp HealthCare systemwide event, a colleague of mine was recognized as a "Pillar Award" winner for leading a diabetes quality management program for poorly controlled diabetic patients. Previously, this physician had flown below the radar, simply doing his job and performing all that was expected of him. His diabetes management program was a passion he had, and it truly made a difference in the quality of care that all of us provided. He was placed on a stage and recognized for the work he had done. The process of visible recognition changed him. He now beams with pride and sees himself differently. He has enthusiastically engaged other system efforts after tasting the opportunity to create change and make a difference. Recognition changes people, changes physicians, replicates behaviors, creates physician loyalty, and builds partnership and trust with a system and its leaders.

Telling an individual that he or she does something well will make that individual better. A friend of mine conducted an unpublished but interesting study that looked at this very issue. He took a random selection of equally educated college students and divided them into three separate groups. A memory recall test was conducted for each group to test how many numbers could be recalled in numerical sequence. The three groups were then randomly separated into "high," "medium," and "low" recall groups (they were not actually separated by performance, but study participants were randomly assigned to each performance group). When the groups came in for a follow-up test, they were "informed" that they were high, average, or below average recallers, and were tested again. The results were revealing. Those who were told that they were "high recallers" became the high recallers by a statistically significant margin. Those who were told they were the "low recallers" became the low recallers. People will do as they believe *they can* do. Recognition can be a change instrument and can improve physician loyalty and performance.

There are a number of methods of "operationalizing" physician recognition. The overarching theme is frequent, visible, and consistent leader effort to simply say "thank you" and "well done." Thanking physicians costs little, builds relationships, improves performance, and changes the tenor of physician relations. Recognizing physicians as a hardwired leader activity can keep physicians loyal and aligned and can sustain behaviors that the system has worked so hard to create.

MANAGING UP

Managing up is the process of positioning others well. At Studer Group, we use managing up as a standard behavioral training tool. Managing up of physicians by staff will change the patient perception of care and will reduce patient anxiety and foster trust with the entire care team. Nursing is considered to be the most trusted of all professions. For example, a treating nurse might say to a patient, "Dr. Jones will be performing your angiogram. He is one of our most experienced and best cardiologists, and his patients just love him. You are in excellent hands." What happens to the patient's perception of the physician and the care team when the most trusted of all professionals says this? Faith in the cardiologist is established, peace of mind is created, anxiety is reduced, and assurance that the patient is in expert hands is affirmed.

The key to leveraging managing up is to transition this effort from an occasional, ad hoc occurrence to a consistent, trained, and executed behavior. Managing up can be applied to every component of the healthcare team. Nurses managing up physicians improve patient perception of physicians. A physician who specifically identifies the expertise of a referral physician builds physician partnership, a sense of team, and quality of care in the eyes of patients.

Managing up happens only if it is trained, expected, and demonstrated by leadership. Managing up happens only if physicians engage in behaviors that are worthy and justify others' speaking well of them. No healthcare team can or should "fake" managing up, and no one should ever say something that isn't true. Managing up should be sincere but strategic in order to position physicians, staff, and the system positively in the eyes of patients.

THANK YOU NOTES

How often does a CEO write a thank you note to a member of the medical staff? This deviates so far from the culture of many systems that the concept and tactic is almost entirely unutilized. How would a medical staff member respond to a handwritten note from a senior system leader to thank him or her for a specific contribution to system efforts? A thank you note as a sincere gesture to physicians changes physician opinion and perception of a system, and can improve physician relationships with leaders.

The most effective thank you notes are ones that are specific. General, non-specific praise is not nearly as effective as targeted and concrete recognition. Thank you notes from senior leaders that are written and sent to the homes of physicians will be something most of the medical staff will have never experienced before and will solidify the opinion that something different and refreshing is happening within the system.

To this day I have a copy of a thank you note written by our system CEO, Mike Murphy, when we began physician training efforts to improve patient satisfaction. This letter made me feel that my work was important and valued by top-tier leadership. Recognition for my efforts kept me going when the prospects of physician change were challenging early in our journey. The best way to diminish ambition, effort, and high performance is to habitually ignore it. Recognition improves effort and performance, and is at the core of the physician engagement process.

RECOGNITION E-MAILS

Though handwritten thank you notes can have impact, electronic communication is what most of us do today. E-mail is a simple and practical means of physician recognition. The value in utilizing e-mail for recognition lies in the ability to transmit the message to people whose opinions matter to the physician. When a physician who is coached improves patient satisfaction performance, send an e-mail to that physician to thank him for his efforts and to acknowledge that those efforts are recognized by patients. More importantly, cc the CEO, medical director, and department chair. Simple recognition transmitted to leadership and physician colleagues promotes coached behaviors, positions change as important, and "illuminates" behavioral improvements for those who may have struggled in the past.

BOOKMARKS

Bookmarks that are used in the outpatient, inpatient, and emergency room environments will recognize physicians, position physicians well to patients, and can serve as physician and organizational marketing tools. Bookmarks can be made for staff physicians, high-volume admitters, hospitalists, and ER physicians. Bookmarks can include a photo of the physician, training, board certifications, special interests, hobbies, and contact information. The best bookmarks will include a personalized statement by the physician that speaks to a philosophy of care, a dedication to quality, and a genuine commitment to what that physician wants to provide to patients.

Bookmarks benefit and recognize physicians through a unique identification of who they are, what they stand for, and a communication and promotion of their commitment to patients. Physician bookmarks allow patients to more easily identify and "promote" physicians involved in their care, particularly in the emergency and inpatient environments.

The key to impacting physicians and patients with bookmarks lies in how the bookmarks are presented by staff as they are given to patients. The point at which the bookmark is provided to the patient is the ideal time to "manage up" physicians. This is also an ideal time to recommunicate contact information that conveys that the system and physician are "here for you" should problems or questions arise after discharge. This is a powerful close to a clinical experience and positions the physician and system as partners dedicated to patients.

PHYSICIAN INVOLVEMENT RECOGNITION

Physician recognition efforts have historically focused on physician clinical or service performance, doing something extraordinary for patients or staff, or community contributions. It is important to broaden recognition criteria to include all activities that leaders want and need other physicians to do. Physician engagement is ultimately defined by physicians' support and involvement in projects, committees, service line development, clinical pathway development, or championing service or quality. Recognize physicians for their contributions to the system. Recognition for involvement will increase involvement. When physician involvement and contributions are well publicized, witnessed by medical staff colleagues, and highly profiled across the system, prospective physician leaders are more apt to embrace additional projects. Place your patient safety committee on the cover of your newsletter, profiling outcomes created by physicians and other team members. Bring in professional photographers, interview them, and tell their stories. Make "rock stars" out of physician high performers and those who have provided guidance and expertise to make the system better.

This public recognition can be applied to a variety of individuals and teams. If you have a group of cardiac surgeons who have achieved high clinical cardiac outcomes, or intensivists and respiratory techs who have "zero" ventilator associated pneumonias, place them as a cover story. Pictures are powerful and make them look good. Create a "buzz" about performance and results. Make others want the same. Place extraordinary outcomes as byproducts of physician involvement, partnership, and leadership.

A PHYSICIAN RECOGNITION BOARD

Dave Fox, the Advocate Good Samaritan CEO, recent recipient of the Fire Starter Hall of Fame Award, and CEO of the year for 2008 by *Hospital Review,* has transformed physician relations and uses frequent and visible recognition strategies to thank physicians for exceptional work. Dave and his team have created a "Recognition Board" for physicians in the lobby of their hospital. The Recognition Board includes a professionally done photo and a description of extraordinary care stories provided by patients. Dave described touching stories of physicians' responses to seeing themselves on the Recognition Board. Dave would see physicians from afar, bringing in their spouses, their parents, and their children to see the Recognition Board. Dave would then send plaques that included the physicians' pictures and stories to the physicians' offices to be placed on the walls of their exam rooms. Interested in disarming physician burnout and cynicism? Try a little public recognition.

OTHER PHYSICIAN RECOGNITION BEST PRACTICES

Studer Group partners have provided extensive experience and best practices from which we frequently learn. Included are physician recognition ideas from systems across the country that have developed and implemented effective physician recognition.

Physician recognition is reflected here in categorical awards tied to organizational values and outcomes that can be used in conjunction with Doctors' Day or any other physician appreciation event. Below are examples that successful organizations have used to recognize and appreciate the medical staff while having some fun in the process.

Categorical Physician Awards:

- Marcus Welby, MD, Award—The doctor with the best patient satisfaction/bedside manner
- Golden Pen Award—The doctor with the best documentation/penmanship
- Dr. McDreamy—The doctor with the most patient recognitions and nominations for excellent care/courtesy/teamwork from staff
- Golden Stethoscope Award—Awarded to the physicians who have the best on-time documentation trends (no late H & Ps, D/C Notes, etc.)
- "Get 'Er Done" Award—Awarded to the doctor with the best timely discharge stats (tied to LOS/Utilization)
- Highest Volume of Direct Admits for the month/quarter/year
- Horizon Award—New physician who demonstrates exemplary clinical practice and physician leadership

An initiative associated with these awards is to assemble a team to interview all physicians who were nominated for the stated categories. Interviewers learn about a physician's likes, personal interests, and what inspires him or her to rise above and do exceptional things. This collected information is then prominently posted in an area within the facility. Seeing the "human" side of medical staff members is a personal way to recognize and appreciate physicians. When a physician's story is told, many new relationships develop as a result of employees and leaders learning about and appreciating the person behind the "MD."

SUMMARY

The absence of physician recognition, even if other good physician collaborative work is done, will leave physicians wondering if anyone knows, cares, realizes, or appreciates what they do. When physicians' work is overlooked, traction for sustained change is diminished, and sustaining the daily effort for system transformation can lose its way. Physician recognition costs almost nothing, makes a difference, and changes physician behavior.

Physician recognition is important enough to improve physician engagement, even if other stages are not executed. It facilitates partnership, creates an environment of collaboration, builds relationships, and raises the "likeability" of the system and its leaders. When recognition is done in collaboration with Stages 1 through 8, a system will have the properties of the best systems anywhere in regard to physician loyalty and partnership.

The journey of physician engagement is about setting the conditions that prompt physicians to jump in, participate, support, and lead the way. Meaningful and genuine physician recognition and appreciation is an irreplaceable leader activity to execute physician engagement.

Key Learnings for Stage 9, "Recognizing Physicians":

1. Physician recognition is historically done with low frequency and effectiveness, even in good systems.
2. Recognition remains a principal predictor of the physician work experience.
3. Physician recognition can improve physician satisfaction, loyalty, and perception of leaders.
4. Recognition of specific physician behaviors will increase the likelihood of those behaviors being repeated.
5. Recognition strategies can include:
   a. Managing up
   b. Thank you notes
   c. E-mail recognition
   d. Bookmarks
   e. Recognition for physician participation and involvement
   f. The Physician Recognition Board
   g. Physician categorical awards
6. Recognition should be frequent, visible, specific, and focused on activities the system needs physicians to do.

The Physician Engagement Leader Checklist

The final pathway and the intent of the stages of this manual are to build an environment that will earn physician loyalty and promote physician partnership to achieve an ambitious organizational vision. In the end, the stages of this manual are about the conditions, experiences, and relationships that drive the complex issue of change and what "flips the switch" for physicians to begin engaging in a system effort. There is clearly no singular strategy that will produce change in well-embedded, longstanding physician attitudes and behaviors. Change drivers must work consistently over time and must impact physicians in a way that shifts perceptions, values, priorities, loyalties, and emotions so that physicians become willing to do something unfamiliar. Change is defined by a personal decision to do things differently and is based upon a choice that is influenced by experiences, circumstances, and relationships. Our approach to physician engagement is about maximizing the probability for change by creating, communicating, and delivering elements of the physician work and personal experiences that will prompt substantive change in most.

Reflect on what has been done, where physician involvement currently stands, and which physician change drivers have, or have not, been activated within the system. Execution of physician engagement is about being comprehensive and deploying strategies that work. Following is a summary leader checklist to execute a strategy of engaging physicians by creating unparalleled partnerships to achieve a shared vision in which patients, physicians, staff, and the organization all win.

PHYSICIAN ENGAGEMENT STAGES WITH SELF-TEST

STAGE 1: Create and Communicate Organizational Vision and Goals: It is not the vision of a system that changes physician behavior; it is how leadership communicates and projects the vision that predicts its impact. "Sharing the playbook" is a *key* responsibility of leadership in creating transformational change, and should precede all other efforts. Physician awareness of vision and goals provides logic, reason, and disclosure of strategies, all of which are requirements for change initiation. In the absence of this deliberate communication, a perfectly sound change effort can fail because physicians may have been uninformed and caught off guard.

The probability of physician support for vision and goals will depend on physician involvement and participation in their creation and launch. Make select physicians of influence "owners" of a strategic plan. What many physicians want more than anything else is to have some control over a clinical environment and input into important decisions. Invite physicians to the table to create, support, and endorse the organization's vision, goals, and strategies, and be prepared to "hear their voices." Physicians' support for a system's effort will depend on the sincerity of leaders' outreach for their expertise, input, and partnership. Proceed only when consensus for vision and goals is achieved, as fractured opinions and intentions between physicians and administrative teams will almost certainly cause an organization to stumble.

Use multi-channel communication and utilize your "owner" physician partners to champion the message. Know that this communication is not subtle, and should be a "drum beat" across the system. Stage 2 should not be engaged until vision and goals are communicated, understood, and supported. Stage 1 should yield a systemwide perception that "something different" is coming and should provide specific clarity as to what that will be.

Stage 1: Create and Communicate Organizational Vision and Goals Leadership Team Checklist:

_______ Create a clear vision for the system that is not a reflection of current operations, but is a clear and specific hope for the future.

_______ Invite select physicians of influence to the table to provide input and approval for a system direction.

_______ Create consensus between physician and administrative leadership so that they speak with a unified voice.

_______ Communicate with medical staff using a shared administration and physician platform with physician leaders serving as the principal communicators in regard to organizational initiatives.

_______ Work in collaboration with physician leadership to create evidence-based goals across pillars.

_______ Communicate vision and goals to the medical staff using multi-channel communication.

STAGE 2: Leadership Development and Accountability for Performance: To engage physicians in organizational change efforts, administrative and physician leaders must have credibility in the eyes of physicians. In order to create organizational credibility, leaders must develop the ability to deliver measurable results across pillars. For leaders to effectively lead and drive outcomes, leaders must be given the skills to lead and they must be held accountable for their performance. Including physician leaders in leadership development and performance accountability will unify the team so that it moves in a singular direction toward shared goals. All leaders, including physician leaders, should be included in leadership development, goal setting, and individual accountability for performance.

Stage 2: Leadership Development and Accountability for Performance Leadership Team Checklist:

_______ Develop quarterly Leadership Development Institutes (LDIs) to provide core leadership skills for the leadership team.

_______ Invite physician leaders to participate in LDIs.

_______ Create and assign weighted "goal sets" for each leader (down to unit managers) that align with system goals.

_______ Establish goals and stretch goals for individual pillars with a five-point graded scale to reflect individual leader performance. Leaders receive a "4" by hitting a goal and a "5" by hitting the stretch goal (this scale can be adjusted).

_______ Create a performance-based leader scorecard containing the leader's assigned goal set.

_______ Leader performance across pillars is tracked in real-time and is transparent to the leadership team.

_______ Share the individual leader accountability model with the general medical staff to convey and project an organizational performance culture.

STAGE 3: Establishing Physician Confidence and Trust: Physician engagement is a "conditional" process. Physicians move forward and align with leaders when specific conditions are met. First, they believe, understand, and support the vision of the system. Second, the leadership team demonstrates a sincere commitment to the physician clinical experience. Third, there is visible, tangible, and consistent responsiveness to physician concerns. Physicians will follow only those whom they trust and will partner only with those they know and believe in. These precursors for physician partnership should be at the core of the organizational mission.

Stage 3: Establishing Physician Confidence and Trust Leadership Team Checklist:

_______ Establish physician satisfaction as part of the pillar-based organizational goals.

_______ Assemble a physician satisfaction team reportable to the CEO with physician satisfaction as an outcome measure.

_______ Establish a physician orientation process to communicate vision, strategy, and goals, and provide physicians with the necessary resources for an efficient practice experience.

_______ Provide personal leader introductions to new physicians, including background, contributions, and personal contact information.

_______ Establish senior leader phone calls to high admitters/key physicians to convey and communicate vision, goals, and efforts underway to improve the physician experience.

_______ Survey physicians to assess physician satisfaction with the clinical experience and interaction with administration.

_______ Develop a priority index of physician issues based on survey feedback.

_______ Deploy communication portals to communicate response to physician issues.

_______ Establish and execute leader rounding on physicians using rounding logs.

_______ Deploy Hourly Rounding. Round on physicians to create awareness of Hourly Rounding and its benefits to patient care.

_______ Deploy Discharge Phone Calls. Round on physicians to create awareness of Discharge Phone Calls.

_______ Implement "Got Chart" as a consistent communication method between physicians and nurses. Round on physicians to create awareness of "Got Chart."

_______ Develop Physician Preference Cards to build familiarity with and the identities of medical staff.

_______ Establish a physician "hotline" to demonstrate leaders' commitment to responsiveness to physician issues.

People will follow those whom they trust, and trust is built on relationships, experiences, and history. Like clarity of vision and goals, this change driver will make or break change efforts for physicians. The absence of trust is mutually exclusive to the physician engagement journey. Physicians will do for leaders what they have seen leaders do for them.

STAGE 4: **Building Physician Leadership:** From the physician perspective, the perception of a physician-led effort changes physician behavior more than an administrative-led effort. Creating and selecting effective physician leaders are key elements to achieving physician engagement. In order for physician leaders to drive organizational performance and support the organizational platform, physician leaders must support organizational efforts, possess the ability to effectively communicate organizational goals and strategies, and be skilled in creating consensus among the general medical staff. Physician leader selection and development and the identification of physician champions will need to be at the core of system efforts.

Stage 4: Building Physician Leadership Team Checklist:

_______ Appoint structural physician leaders who possess attributes consistent with the character and vision of the organization.

_______ Create consensus between the executive team and structural physician leadership on vision, goals, and strategy.

_______ Include physicians in leadership development curriculum.

_______ Select physician champions according to selection criteria.

_______ Create clear outcome goals for physician champions.

_______ Create a physician champion contract that specifies time requirements, pay, objectives, and reportability.

_______ Train and develop physician champions.

_______ Communicate the role of the physician champions systemwide so that the medical staff are aware of their purposes and goals.

STAGE 5: Training Physicians: The training and development of physicians as an organizational objective will make physicians better clinicians, and can create greater consistency in how physicians treat patients, staff, and each other. Training is never delivered in the spirit of manipulating physician conduct to achieve a system agenda, but rather is intended to help physicians become more successful by deploying behaviors that work. How physicians treat patients, staff, and each other are coachable behaviors, and will have a significant influence on the culture and performance of a system. Coaching and "investing" in physicians, when done expertly by trained, supported, and activated champions, clarifies the physician role in a system committed to clinical and service excellence.

Stage 5: Training Physicians Leadership Team Checklist:

_______ Design a sequenced curriculum to be delivered by physician champions or external physician trainers.

_______ Create and arrange a "launch event" as a CME activity. Invite affiliated physicians and incentivize or "require" attendance for employed physicians.

_______ Create medical staff "buy-in" and *make the case* for change using compelling industry evidence that is important to physicians.

_______ Create a "burning platform" using internal performance data. Create true urgency and relevance for change efforts.

_______ Train clinical physicians to use AIDET.

_______ Develop an ongoing training method to sustain physician awareness and development of behaviors that are consistent with the organizational performance and service culture.

STAGE 6: Physician Measurement and Balanced Scorecards: Properly applied physician performance assessment and reporting to physicians are core strategies that align physician behavior to achieve pillar goals. Feedback and physician knowledge of their own performance as compared to peers and goals intensifies physician effort and focuses behaviors. Measurement creates the burning platform, the need for change, clarity of current performance, tracking of improvement, and a performance culture. Well-executed physician performance reporting can be one of the most powerful drivers of physician behavioral change.

Stage 6: Physician Measurement and Balanced Scorecards Leadership Team Checklist:

_______ Create specific performance goals for physicians across pillars, with input from physician leadership. Individual physician goals should be aligned with organizational goals.

_______ Communicate specific goals to physicians.

_______ Develop a physician scorecard to assess and report physician performance across pillars.

_______ Create a reporting method in which physicians can see results across pillars as a *comparative* measurement. Consider transparency of physician performance as physicians become accustomed to performance assessment and reporting.

_______ Deploy physician champions to assist physicians who consistently fall below goal expectations.

_______ Implement an incentive system for employed or contracted physicians who achieve pillar goals.

STAGE 7: **Implementing Physician Behavioral Standards:** The articulation and communication of a code of conduct that communicates behavioral expectations can change and align physician behavior. Like all other change strategies, the impact of this strategy depends entirely on how it is positioned and communicated by leadership. If a code of conduct is positioned as important, then it will be seen as important. Consistency of behaviors is at the core of system change, and consistency of behaviors requires the communication of what those behaviors entail. Physicians are less likely to engage in troublesome behavior if a code of conduct is developed, communicated, trained, and supported by respected physician leaders as a clear systemwide commitment to safety, quality, and service.

Stage 7: Implementing Physician Behavioral Standards Leadership Team Checklist:

_______ Select a team of physicians to draft a code of conduct.

_______ Review Joint Commissions Behavioral Standards criteria for elements to include in a code of conduct.

_______ Create a list of desired and prohibited behaviors that are consistent with the vision, values, and culture of the organization.

_______ Create a code of conduct to include how physicians treat staff, patients, and colleagues.

_______ Communicate the code of conduct to the medical staff using physician leadership and respected clinicians who assisted in drafting the behavioral standards.

_______ Use the code of conduct for physician orientation and training.

_______ Require physicians to sign the code of conduct during privileging or recredentialing.

_______Create a consistent response strategy for code of conduct violations that is included in updated bylaws.

STAGE 8: Managing the Disruptive Physician: Leaders' responses to violations of the code of conduct are ultimately a measure of the depth of leaders' true commitment to change. The consequences of unmanaged physician behaviors can have far-reaching organizational impact and demand leader action. A response strategy to disruptive physician behavior must be consistent, fair, and proactive. If there is not visible management of physician behaviors that are counter to the mission of the organization, the credibility of the mission will be called into doubt.

Stage 8: Managing the Disruptive Physician Leadership Team Checklist:

_______ Update by-laws to create a consistent response to disruptive behaviors.

_______ Intervene consistently when the code of conduct is violated.

_______ Stratify disruptive behaviors as singular or recurrent.

_______ Designate structural physician leaders to have "awareness" and "intervention" conversations with disruptive physicians.

_______ Contract third-party resources to assist disruptive physicians, if necessary.

_______ Enact a re-entry policy and conditions for physicians who undergo a third-party intervention.

STAGE 9: **Recognizing Physicians:** Physician recognition replicates and propagates physician behaviors. Leveraging the influence of recognition as a systemwide effort improves physicians' relationships with leaders and verifies the system's value of physician efforts. Recognition costs little, impacts behavior, and can build relationships that are at the heart of physician partnership, collaboration, and engagement.

Stage 9: Recognizing Physicians Leadership Team Checklist:

_______ Train staff and physicians on how to "manage up."

_______ Write personal thank-you notes to physicians regarding specific activities that represent the values and character of the organization.

_______ Use email to recognize physician performance. These emails can be sent in real-time and cc'ed to senior leadership.

_______ Use bookmarks to profile and manage up physicians to patients.

_______ Use high-profile physician recognition efforts, such as physician photographs and stories of extraordinary care in the hospital lobby.

_______ Thank and recognize physicians for participation in and contribution to system efforts.

_______ Create a categorical, physician-specific award system that can cycle through the organization. Make physician award efforts high-profile, meaningful, and fun.

The Heart of Change

"The strongest principle of growth lies in human choice."
—George Eliot

Do Stages 1 through 9 guarantee physician engagement? No, not for everyone. Rarely, though, is "everyone" necessary to transform an organization and change its culture. Most often, extraordinary change is led by a small, unified group of passionate, relentless, intense leaders who are at the core who bring about change by inspiring others. Great leaders are rarely driven by strategy alone. Great leaders gather and inspire others to look beyond themselves to a higher, unifying cause dedicated to changing lives, caring for others, lifting spirits, curing disease, relieving pain, wiping tears, and unleashing all that medicine should be. This manual is about breaking barriers and releasing the pause in the physicians' minds that cynicism and exhaustion can build.

I recently spoke with a colleague who is a practicing internist and leads a local medical group. He told me a story of his nephew who wanted to be a physician from a very young age. He described his young nephew as having a "calling" to practice medicine. He told me that his nephew would go on rounds, take house calls with him, and was steadfast in his commitment to become a physician.

While in college, this young man began to have a change of heart, and thought an MBA might be a better option. He called his uncle and broke the news. His physician uncle asked him to come to his home since they lived close to each other. When his nephew arrived, his uncle brought him to his study, handed him an old shoebox, and said to him, "Take a look at these." He left his nephew alone, and closed the door behind him.

My colleague returned nearly an hour later. His nephew was on his knees and had spread hundreds of cards over the floor of the study, reading each of them. He looked up from reading the notes patients had written to his uncle with tears in his eyes. "I am going to be a physician." That was all he said. And so he did.

What drives the physician is no different from what drives the human spirit. It is the heart and the emotions that change what we do more than anything. This book is meant to guide leaders and systems toward reconnecting physicians to the place that so many have lost. This is our life, and we have worked too hard to miss what is standing right in front of us, shrouded by workload, regulation, personal struggles, and the disillusion that somehow medicine should be more than what we have today. I am saddened to know that nearly 60 percent of practicing physicians would not choose this profession again. What did we do to come to this? Perhaps we have taken our eyes off of the patient and have become distracted by the circumstances around us.

It is not too late. The decision to renew, refocus, rededicate, and practice what we hoped to have is here to take. It is a matter of choice. A fulfilled life is elusive and invisible, but you know for sure when you have it. Take it. It is behind the door of every exam room. It is at the bedside with the family of a dying grandfather. It is with the adolescent whom you counsel on smoking. It is with the worried preschool teacher who has a self-limited pharyngitis and who is seeing you again. It is with the high school baseball coach with new onset diabetes. It is with the 48-year-old with metastatic cancer who is losing his fight, and comes to you to tell him the truth. It is with the wife who cries over the death of her 52-year-old husband whom she lost from complications of his alcoholism. This is one day. This was my today.

We work diligently and faithfully to improve healthcare performance by deploying tactics and strategies. If only creating change were that simple. Real transformation requires a much greater force. True change is powered by the soul and by an inherent human desire to make something better, to feel assured and resolved about what we have chosen to do. We want to see ourselves as people who consider the values and welfare of others above ourselves. We want to believe in what we do, and to fill an elusive void with fairness, compassion, honesty, empathy, and caring. We have better lives when we live better lives. We have better lives when we see beyond personal pursuits to a more important cause—to make a difference, to contribute, to make something better, to do the right thing, and to change lives.

The intention of this manual is to help leaders and physicians come together to care for the patient above all else, and to make the pursuit of extraordinary care, saving lives, and making a difference our shared purpose. When leaders and physicians become guided by a collaborative vision and unified effort, with physicians at the lead and champions for change, your organization can become unstoppable. Let's get to work and get this done.

Bibliography

[1] American Heart Association. Department of Veteran Affairs.

[2] Press Ganey. "Patient Satisfaction and Physicians Satisfaction Correlation Report." 2006.

[3] Physician Press Ganey Associates, Inc. "Physician Perspectives on American Hospitals." *Hospital Check-Up Report,* 2007.

[4] Bursell, Amy L., Lyn Ketelsen, and Christine M. Meade. "Effects of Nursing Rounds on Patients' Call Light Use, Satisfaction, and Safety." *American Journal of Nursing* 106, no. 9 (2006): 58-70.

[5] Bates, David, et al. "The Incidence and Severity of Adverse Events Affecting Patients After Discharge from the Hospital." *Annals of Internal Medicine* 138 (2003): 161-74.

[6] Engel, Kirsten G., et al. "Patient Comprehension of Emergency Department Care and Instructions: Are Patients Aware of When They Do Not Understand?" *Annals of Emergency Medicine* 53 (2008): 454-61.

[7] Physician Communication Skills Survey. 2001.

[8] Chang, John T., et al. "Patient Global Ratings of Their Health Care Are Not Correlated with the Technical Quality of Their Care." *Annals of Internal Medicine* 144, (2006): 665-72.

[9] Engstrom, S. and D. J. Madlon-Kay. "Choosing a Family Physician: What Do Patients Want to Know?" *Minnesota Medicine* 81, no.12 (1998): 22-6.

[10] American Hospital Association. "American Hospital Association Reality Check II." 1998.

[11] Harris, Lisa E., Richard S. Kurz, and Koichiro Otani. "Managing Primary Care Using Patient Satisfaction Measures." *Journal of Healthcare Management* 50, no. 5 (2005): 311-24.

[12] Harris, Lisa E., Richard S. Kurz, and Koichiro Otani. "Managing Primary Care Using Patient Satisfaction Measures." *Journal of Healthcare Management* 50, no. 5 (2005): 311-24.

[13] Wiebe, C. "What Did You Say? Tips for Talking More Clearly to Patients." *ACP Observer*, December 1997.

[14] Phillips, A., C. Vincent, and M. Young. "Why Do People Sue Doctors? A Study of Patients and Relatives Taking Legal Action." *Lancet* 343 (1994): 1609-13.

[15] Gonzalez, M. L. and E. J. Slora. "Medical Professional Liability Claims and Premiums, 1985-1989." In *Socioeconomic Characteristics of Medical Practice*, ed. M. Gonzalez, (Chicago: American Medical Association, 1990/1991), 15-20.

[16] O'Daniel, M. and A. Rosenstein. "Disruptive Behavior and Clinical Outcomes: Perceptions of Nurses and Physicians." *Nursing Management* 2005, 18-29.

[17] Green, Marianne, Gregory Makoul, and Amanda Zick. "An Evidence-Based Perspective on Greetings in Medical Encounters." *Archives of Internal Medicine* 167 (2007): 1172-76.

[18] Beale, E., et al. "Impact of Physician Sitting Versus Standing During Inpatient Oncology Consultations: Patients' Preference and Perception of Compassion and Duration." *Journal of Pain and Symptom Management* 29, no. 5 (2005): 489-97.

[19] Green, M., G. Makuos, and A. Zick. "An Evidence-Based Perspective on Greetings in Medical Encounters." *Archives of Internal Medicine* 167 (2007): 1172-76.

[20] Child, Stephen, et al. "How Many Health Professionals Does a Patient See During an Average Hospital Stay?" *Journal of the New Zealand Medical Association* 120, no. 1253 (2007).

[21] Press Ganey. "Medical Practice Pulse Report." 2006.

[22] Hays, Ron D., et al. "Physician Communication When Prescribing New Medications." *Archives of Internal Medicine* 166 (2006): 1855-62.

[23] *Mayo Clinic Proceedings* 80, no. 8 (2005): 991-94.

[24] Blue Cross Quality Health Care Report Card. 2006, 2007 and 2008.

[25] Weber, D. O. "Poll Results: Doctors' Disruptive Behavior Disturbs Physician Leaders." *Physician Executive*, September-October 2004, 6-14.

[26] American Medical Association. "Physicians with Disruptive Behavior." CEJA Report 106.

[27] Pfifferling, J. H. "Managing the Unmanageable Physician." *Family Practice Management*, November-December 1997, 76-92.

[28] Weber, D. O. "For Safety's Sake Disruptive Behavior Must Be Tamed." *Physician Executive*, September-October 2004, 16-17.

[29] Youssi, M. D. "JCAHO Standards Help Address Disruptive Physician Behavior." *Physician Executive*, November-December 2002, 12-13.

[30] Mareiniss, D. P. "Decreasing GME Training Stress to Foster Residents' Professionalism." *Academic Medicine* 79 (2004): 825-31.

[31] Rosenstein, A. "Nurse-Physician Relationships: Impact on Nurse Satisfaction and Retention." *American Journal of Nursing* 102, no. 6 (2002): 26-34.

[32] Glasscock, Sue, and Kimberly Gram. "Winning Ways: Establishing an Effective Workplace Recognition System." *National Productivity Review* 14, no. 3 (2001): 91-102.

Resources

Accelerate the momentum of your Healthcare Flywheel[SM].

Visit www.studergroup.com/engagingphysicians to access and download many of the resources, examples, and tools mentioned in *Engaging Physicians.*

ARTICLES

"Keep Your Patients Coming Back"
MGMA Connexion—August 2008
by: Quint Studer

BLOGS

"Achieving Physician Engagement and Collaboration"
by: Wolfram Schynoll, M.D., FACEP,
Studer Group Medical Director and Physician Coach

To read related articles and blogs, visit www.studergroup.com or visit www.studergroup.com/engagingphysicians for more information on the resources listed above.

BOOKS

Practicing Excellence—So much of a medical organization's success rides on the leadership, conduct, and performance of its physicians. How does a healthcare organization engage its physicians to lead by example? And how does a physician do what needs to be done to foster satisfaction and loyalty among patients? *Practicing Excellence*, written by Stephen C. Beeson, M.D., eloquently answers these questions.

Hardwiring Excellence—Quint Studer helps healthcare professionals to rekindle the flame and offers a road map to creating and sustaining a Culture of Service and Operational Excellence that drives bottom-line results.

Leadership and Medicine—Floyd D. Loop, M.D., retired chief executive of the Cleveland Clinic, gives readers a compelling inside look at what it takes to run a major medical system and teaches readers valuable lessons about the art and science of leadership.

For more information about these books or to view additional books, visit www.firestarterpublishing.com.

WEBINAR TRACKS

Engaging Physicians
Presented by Stephen Beeson, M.D.

Dealing with "Special" Colleagues: Discouraging Disruptive Behavior
Presented by Gerald Hickson, M.D., Faculty, Vanderbilt University Medical Center

Physician Accountability—Aligning Physician Performance with Organizational Goals to Drive Clinical and Financial Outcomes
Presented by Wolf Schynoll, M.D., FACEP

For more information on Studer Group's Webinar Tracks, visit www.studergroup.com/webinars.

SOFTWARE SOLUTIONS AND DVD TRAINING RESOURCES

Leader Evaluation Manager™
Results Through Focus and Accountability
Studer Group's Leader Evaluation Manager is a web-based application that automates the goal setting and performance review process for all leaders, while ensuring that the performance metrics of individual leaders are aligned with the overall goals of the organization.

Building Patient Trust with AIDET® Training DVD
Built in partnership with Vanderbilt University Medical Center and Studer Group, the Building Patient Trust with AIDET training DVD is ideal for training staff, leaders, and physician groups on how to use the key communication steps of AIDET: Acknowledge, Introduce, Duration, Explanation and Thank You. Participants will learn the what, why, and how of reducing patient anxiety, improving clinical outcomes, and creating a better patient experience with AIDET.

For more information on Studer Group Solutions or DVD Training Resources, visit www.studergroup.com.

INSTITUTES

Studer Group Institutes offer a range of learning opportunities for health care organizations beginning their journey to implementing a Culture of Excellence and those looking to create change in a specific area.

Taking You and Your Organization to the Next Level
At this two-day institute, leaders learn tactics proven to help them quickly move results in the most critical areas: HCAHPS, Core Measures, preventable readmissions, hospital-acquired conditions, and more. They walk away with a clear action plan that yields measurable improvement within 90 days. Even more important, they learn how to implement these tactics in the context of our Evidence-Based Leadership framework so they can execute quickly and consistently and sustain the results over time.

Excellence in the Emergency Department: Hardwiring Flow & Patient Experience
Crowded Emergency Departments and long patient wait times are no longer acceptable, especially with public reporting of data in the near future. We can predict with great accuracy when lulls and peak times will be, and we know exactly how to improve flow and provide better quality care. This institute will reveal a few simple, hard-hitting tactics that solve the most pressing ED problems and create better clinical quality and patient perception of care throughout the entire hospital stay.

The Physician Partnership Institute: A Path to Alignment, Engagement and Integration
The changes mandated by health reform make it clear: There will surely be some sort of "marriage" between hospitals and physicians. Regardless of what form it takes, we must start laying the groundwork for a rewarding partnership now. Learn our

comprehensive methodology for getting physicians aligned with, engaged in, and committed to your organization so that everyone is working together to provide the best possible clinical care, improve HCAHPS results, increase patient loyalty, and gain market share.

What's Right in Health Care®
One of the largest healthcare peer-to-peer learning conferences in the nation, What's Right in Health Care brings organizations together to share ideas that have been proven to make healthcare better. Thousands of leaders attend this institute every year to network with their peers, to hear top industry experts speak, and to learn tactical best practices that allow them to accelerate and sustain performance.

For information on Continuing Education Credits, visit www.studergroup.com/cmecredits.

TOOLKITS

Physician Collaboration Toolkit
This is a guide for administrators and other healthcare professionals to collaborate with physicians. Only an electronic version format of this toolkit is available at no charge to Studer Group Partner Organizations.

Physician Selection Toolkit
This toolkit offers a clear-cut strategy for hiring physicians who have both clinical competence and strong interpersonal skills. Only an electronic version format is offered. This toolkit is available at no charge to Studer Group Partner Organizations.

For more information on toolkits, visit www.studergroup.com.

ABOUT STUDER GROUP

Studer Group's mission is to change the face of healthcare by creating a better place for employees to work, physicians to practice medicine, and patients to receive care. Studer Group is an outcomes-based healthcare performance improvement firm that coaches hundreds of hospitals, health systems, medical practices, and end-of life organizations to achieve and sustain clinical results. To learn more about Studer Group, visit www.studergroup.com.

Visit www.studergroup.com/engagingphysicians to access and download many of the resources, examples, and tools mentioned in *Engaging Physicians.*

Acknowledgments

Quint Studer—For making physician engagement a central effort in Studer Group and relentlessly pushing all of us to continually improve.

BG Porter—For his early readership and support when Engaging Physicians was in its first version.

Bekki Kennedy—For making this book happen, and giving me the freedom and opportunity to precisely convey the spirit of this manual.

Mel Loughnane—For being a great friend and an effective, brutally honest reviewer of the first manuscript.

Mom and Dad—For always supporting me, even when I made questionable choices very early in my life.

Donald Balfour, MD—The leader of Sharp Rees-Stealy and whose support for the Sharp Experience changed everything.

Dottie DeHart—A professional editor who let me write freely but kept the manuscript disciplined.

Julie Kennedy, RN—For her expert professional and personal guidance.

Jay Kaplan, MD—For teaching me how to present to others and sharing his intellectual materials.

Wolf Schynoll, MD—For providing great input on the early manuscript to make it better.

Dave Fox—A visionary leader who represents the best there is in building physician partnership, for his invaluable input on the manuscript.

Ken Davis—For his insightful review of the manuscript and his passionate leadership at North Miss and San Antonio.

Barbara Paul, MD—For her early input on the "free write" version and her dedication to physician partnership.

Sandy Burstein—For his valued suggestions and the extraordinary example he sets for all physician leaders.

Bill Soto, MD—For enduring a pre-first version of the initial manuscript.

Henry Veldman—For his detailed review and prompt feedback between the first and second versions.

Sherry Gentry—For her readership of the manuscript and her appreciation of the importance and challenges in engaging physicians.

Kelly Dickey—For doing everything behind the scenes and making sure I am in the right place at the right time, every time.

About Dr. Beeson

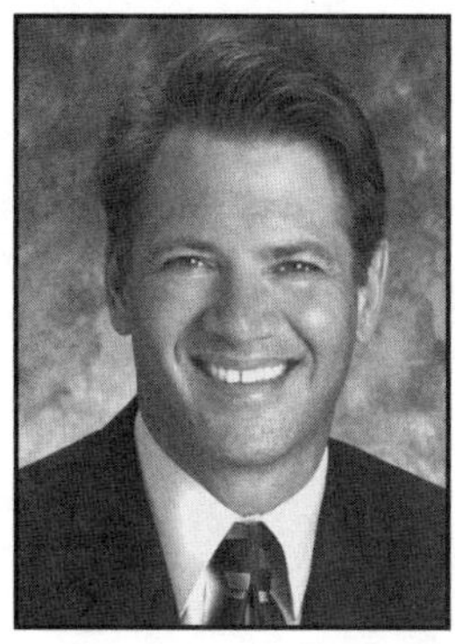

Dr. Stephen Beeson is a nationally recognized speaker who has provided tools and tactics for engaging and training physicians to hundreds of medical groups and hospitals and thousands of physicians throughout the country. In September of 2006, Dr. Beeson released his book Practicing Excellence: A Physician's Manual to Exceptional Health Care. This national bestseller articulates a strategic, prescriptive, "how-to" approach to engage and train physicians to drive organizational performance.

Stephen Beeson is a board-certified family medicine physician practicing with Sharp Rees-Stealy Medical Group. In 2002, Dr. Beeson was selected by Sharp HealthCare leadership to serve as the physician fire starter for the Sharp Experience, an organizational commitment to service and operational excellence. Dr. Beeson's patient satisfaction ranks him in the 99th percentile nationwide, and the San Diego County Medical Society voted him as one of San Diego's Best Physicians in 2005, 2006, 2007, and 2008. Recently, Dr. Beeson was a recipient of the Center of Recognized Excellence Award for Individual Service Excellence, and Sharp HealthCare was the recipient of the prestigious Malcolm Baldrige Award for 2007 for organizational performance.

Dr. Beeson graduated magna cum laude from the University of California, where he also completed his medical school and residency training.

Dr. Beeson has authored, developed, and implemented physician training programs including the Sharp Rees-Stealy Physician Pledge, the Physician Performance Dashboard for patient satisfaction, the Physician Guide to Service Excellence, the Physician Excellence Award Program, new physician orientation and training, individual physician coaching, physician interviewing and selection processes, and the Acts of Excellence electronic physician training program. Dr. Beeson now brings these proven tactics to medical groups and medical staffs across the country.

Dr. Beeson is passionate about providing exceptional care to patients and works with Studer Group as a medical advisor, speaker, and physician coach to broaden the difference he can make with physicians across the country.

Index

Q

R

HOW TO ORDER ADDITIONAL COPIES OF

Engaging Physicians:
A Manual to Physician Partnership

Orders may be placed:

Online at:
www.firestarterpublishing.com
www.studergroup.com

By phone at: 866-354-3473

By mail at: Fire Starter Publishing
913 Gulf Breeze Parkway, Suite 6
Gulf Breeze, FL 32561

(Bulk discounts are available.)

Engaging Physicians is also available online at
www.amazon.com